Autism Missed and Misdiagnosed

by the same author

**A Guide to Mental Health Issues in Girls and Young
Women on the Autism Spectrum**
Diagnosis, Intervention and Family Support
Judy Eaton
ISBN 978 1 78592 092 9
eISBN 978 1 78450 355 0

of related interest

Autism and Masking
How and Why People Do It, and the Impact It Can Have
Felicity Sedgwick, Dr. Laura Hull and Helen Ellis
ISBN 978 1 78775 579 6
eISBN 978 1 78775 580 2

Taking Off the Mask
**Practical Exercises to Help Understand and Minimise
the Effects of Autistic Camouflaging**
Hannah Louise Belcher
ISBN 978 1 78775 589 5
eISBN 978 1 78775 590 1

Understanding Pathological Demand Avoidance Syndrome in Children
A Guide for Parents, Teachers and Other Professionals
Phil Christie, Margaret Duncan, Zara Healy and Ruth Fidler
ISBN 978 1 84905 074 6
eISBN 978 0 85700 253 2

Autism Missed and **Misdiagnosed**

IDENTIFYING, UNDERSTANDING AND SUPPORTING DIVERSE AUTISTIC IDENTITIES

Dr Judy Eaton

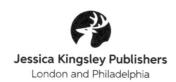

Jessica Kingsley Publishers
London and Philadelphia

First published in Great Britain in 2024 by Jessica Kingsley Publishers
An imprint of John Murray Press

I

Content Warning: This book mentions abuse, anxiety, bipolar disorder, bullying, death,
depression, eating disorders, hospitalisation, rape, self-harm, suicide and trauma.

A CIP catalogue record for this title is available from the
British Library and the Library of Congress

ISBN 978 1 83997 460 1
eISBN 978 1 83997 461 8

Printed and bound in Great Britain by CPI Group

Jessica Kingsley Publishers' policy is to use papers that are natural,
renewable and recyclable products and made from wood grown in
sustainable forests. The logging and manufacturing processes are expected
to conform to the environmental regulations of the country of origin.

Jessica Kingsley Publishers
Carmelite House
50 Victoria Embankment
London EC4Y 0DZ

www.jkp.com

John Murray Press
Part of Hodder & Stoughton Limited
An Hachette UK Company

Acknowledgements

This book has been written at the end of a long and interesting career as a psychologist and reflects the many challenges that face autistic people that I have witnessed over the years working in a variety of settings.

I have been overwhelmed by the honesty of the many contributors who have told their personal stories. Some of these stories are hard to read, and, sadly, not all result in a positive outcome. I would like to personally thank every one of these autistic women whom I have got to know either as clients or colleagues, and some of whom I now proudly count as my friends.

I would also like to thank the brave parents who were kind enough to allow me to share their stories, including Jeremy and Jane, and not forgetting the wonderful Paula who has fought tirelessly to ensure that the Oliver McGowan training in autism is now mandatory.

I dedicate this book to the amazing young lady whose story is told in the final chapter, and who, at the time of writing, is still in hospital; to Oliver and Ayla who are sadly no longer here to tell their stories; and last, but not least, to my own son David, who was autistic and who lost his life at the age of 35, due in no small part to a lack of understanding on the part of doctors who treated him. David was the reason I began work in this area and remains the inspiration and motivation for this book.

Contents

CHAPTER ONE

Overview of the Diagnostic Process for Autism in the UK

This chapter will provide an overview of the diagnostic process for autism spectrum conditions, discussing the diagnostic manuals and criteria. It will also explore concepts such as controversial diagnostic formulations such as the pathological (or extreme) demand avoidant (PDA) profile and will explain the differences between this and other diagnoses such as conduct disorder, oppositional defiant disorder (ODD) and antisocial personality disorder. The issue of girls, in particular, being diagnosed with emotionally unstable personality disorder (EUPD) will also be discussed.

In an ideal world a book like this would not need to exist. In early discussions about it, the title was discussed at length, and it was initially suggested that we include the words 'complex' and 'perplexing' in the title, as this is how individuals are often referred to. However, it was decided that these descriptions were, at best, mildly derogatory towards the autistic community. Complex and perplexing suggest a deficit model: that individuals are somehow difficult or challenging. However, the original title of the book was initially chosen to reflect the perceptions of many clinicians working in both Child and Adolescent Mental Health Services (CAMHS) and adult mental health services, not to mention medical and social work professionals. It has become much more pertinent in recent times following the publication of the

Royal College of Paediatrics and Child Health (RCPCH) perplexing presentations (PP)/fabricated or induced illness (FII) in children guidance published in March 2021 (RCPCH 2021). Whilst these guidelines highlight the challenges of identifying cases where parents may deliberately induce illness or fabricate illness in their child, more worrying from an autistic point of view, the guidelines also include descriptions of parents of children with 'perplexing presentations'. Basically, under these guidelines, any parent who (a) seeks multiple assessments of a child by different professionals/insists upon a second opinion, (b) has a child where the difficulties are not seen in contexts other than the family home or (c) is unable/unwilling to ensure that the child attends school and has access to a social life could potentially be flagged up as an FII case. Sadly, this description fits many undiagnosed autistic children and puts them and their family at risk of being dragged through long and incredibly traumatic investigations of their lifestyle and parenting and, in some tragic cases, having their child removed. There is currently only anecdotal and limited evidence available regarding exactly how many families with diagnosed or undiagnosed autistic children have faced this situation. Colleagues working in legal and social work teams certainly report a growing number of cases. This issue is discussed more fully in Chapters Eight and Nine, from a personal and professional perspective.

The issue of 'complex' young people has also been at the heart of work carried out since 2019 (completed in March 2023) by the Strategic Oversight Board chaired by the (then) Children's Commissioner Anne Longfield. This was set up to examine and question the improvement programme implemented by NHS England and which aimed to improve outcomes for young people with learning difficulties and autism detained under the Mental Health Act in adolescent inpatient services across the country. This group has led to the establishment of other, specialised task force groups. One in particular was set up specifically to look at the critical issue of a number of highly complex children, many of whom are autistic, for whom appropriate support has proved challenging. It is likely that there could be several hundred children who fall into this category and who are currently supported in a range of settings from inpatient units, through to residential care homes, secure children's homes and youth offending institutions.

I worked for several years in inpatient services and was invited to become part of these groups. During my time in the sector, I was shocked and surprised to note just how many autistic children were detained in hospital. Some were already diagnosed, many were not, and were often described as 'complex' because they did not easily fit any known, or well understood, diagnostic category. Very often they had been given a variety of labels ranging from conduct disorder and ODD through to EUPD. One young person, 'Bethany', was detained for over two years in a hospital that struggled to manage her complex needs. She is autistic, with a PDA profile. For a shockingly long time, she was placed in a small seclusion room without any company or stimulation and was fed through a hatch in the door. Now, thanks to a concerted and hard-fought campaign by her father, she is placed in bespoke provision and is no longer presenting with the degree of 'challenging' behaviour that was reported to have necessitated secluding her in this way. Bethany's full story is outlined in Chapter Eleven. As a clinician specialising now in 'complex' presentations, I know that Bethany's story is by no means unique. There are many children and young people both in hospital and in the community where they and their families are experiencing high levels of distress, and no one appears willing or able to support them. There are very few specialist community teams, and therapeutic and parental support is often non-existent or subject to an excessively long wait. The Independent Oversight Board has also highlighted that many young people in hospitals still do not have access to a thorough assessment by experts in 'complex' or 'perplexing' presentations.

Part of the problem seems to be because many diagnostic teams in the United Kingdom are, and have been for some time, overwhelmed by the sheer volume of referrals they have received. I was the lead clinician in an NHS diagnostic team in the United Kingdom which was set up in 2002. At this time, it was anticipated that we would receive between 40 and 60 referrals per year. By the time I left the team in 2011 we were regularly receiving in excess of 360 referrals per year. My successor in the team recently reported that referrals are currently around 600 per year.

The prevalence rate in the UK for autism in 2014 (Rogers *et al.* 2014) was reported to be 1.7 per cent, and the US the most recent CDC figures

(Johns Hopkins University 2020) suggested that 1:36 children (2.8 per cent) had a diagnosis of autism.

Various reasons have been proposed for this increase. A study by Gillberg and Wing in 2007 cited early prevalence estimates of less than one in two thousand children. However, it was clear that this estimate was more than likely based upon Kanner's (1943) original diagnostic criteria. Suggestions about why there has been this apparent increase range from greater awareness of the breadth and dimensional nature of what has come to be referred to as the 'autism spectrum' (Baron-Cohen *et al.* 2009; Kogan *et al.* 2009; Zaroff and Uhm 2011) through to possible environmental factors (Russell and Kelly 2011).

Whatever the reason it is hardly surprising that diagnostic teams are struggling to assess and diagnose all of the children who are referred in a timely manner. A recent survey by the UK charity Ambitious about Autism found that many of the 4000 parents surveyed reported that they had waited up to three years for an assessment. In addition, it is not always possible for either generic CAMHS or specialist neurodevelopmental teams to follow the National Institute for Care and Clinical Excellence (NICE) guidelines for the assessment and diagnosis of autism spectrum disorders in under 19s (NICE 2017), due to the sheer volume of referrals they face. The NICE guidelines recommend that assessments are carried out by a multidisciplinary team (including a combination of psychiatrist, paediatrician, clinical psychologists, speech and language therapists and/ or occupational therapists). Information should also be gathered from parents, from standardised assessments and from a third party, such as school. In reality, many referrals are initially screened (or 'triaged') by a variety of professionals with differing levels of expertise. Some assessments are carried out by a single professional. This often means that any child or young person who presents as 'atypical', or who does not fit into any well-understood diagnostic category, may not be put forward for further assessment. Their family is often left to struggle on as best they can, and ultimately the child becomes even more 'complex'.

Aside from the issue of having to wait for an assessment, it appears that, despite much awareness raising, there are still a number of professionals who remain less than well informed about the multitude of ways in which an autistic person may present.

This may be due, in part, to hypotheses such as Simon Baron-Cohen's (Baron-Cohen 2002) 'Extreme Male Brain' theory. Baron-Cohen theorised that there are a number of stereotypically 'male' characteristics that include better visuo-spatial awareness, later language development in male infants and less well-developed social skills. He further explored the idea that these traits are more apparent in autistic males and used this theory to hypothesise that autism may reflect an 'extreme' male brain.

At this time, the male to female ratio for autism was reported as being around four males to every one female, and even as late as the 2018 CDC data, it continued to be reported that there is a significant gender difference in the prevalence rate of autism with 1 in 34 boys compared to 1 in 145 girls. This is despite the fact that it has become increasingly apparent that there are many autistic females, and the way that they present does not always fit this stereotypical pattern.

Added to this, although there is scant formal research about it, are the number of autistic individuals who either identify as non-binary or transgender. This ultimately means that using diagnostic criteria that are likely to miss any person who does not fit neatly into the 'male' version of autism is likely to result in many either being misdiagnosed, or missed altogether. It is important to stress at this point that there are a number of biological female autistics who do present in a more stereotypical manner, and as many biological males who present in, what has come to be known as, a more 'female' autistic way. This is before considering those who identify as non-binary or agender, who may not fit either pattern.

Unfortunately, many of the tools and screening questionnaires that have historically been used in autism assessments rely quite heavily upon the stereotypical and more traditionally 'male' diagnostic criteria.

The ADI-R, for example, was originally developed in 1989 and was initially designed as a research, rather than as a diagnostic, tool. In 1994, Lord, Rutter and LeCouteur revised the tool and produced the ADI-R. Questions in the ADI-R focus on communication and language skills, including speech development, appropriate use of language and the ability to maintain a conversation. It also has a 'social interaction' section which examines how the individual interacts with others, interprets emotional responses and is able to show emotion. Finally, it examines stereotyped behaviour, fixation upon unusual items, hand flapping and other repetitive movements.

The AQ-10 (Allison, Auyeung and Baron-Cohen 2012) is a questionnaire which is freely available to download and is frequently used as an initial screen when adults, in particular, are seeking a diagnosis. It is quick and easy to complete. However, the male bias in this particular questionnaire is clear in statements such as: 'I like to collect information about categories of things (e.g., types of cars, types of bird, types of train, types of plant etc.)' (p.1).

Even the ADOS (Autism Diagnostic Observation Schedule) (Gotham *et al.* 2006), which is a tool used to examine play and social interaction in children and imagination and social interaction in adults, is fairly male centric as it includes evaluation of reciprocal conversation, eye contact and prosody (tone of voice), all of which can be significantly less obviously impaired in most females, some males and non-binary individuals. The issue of misdiagnosis will be discussed more fully in Chapter Two.

Autism and ADHD

Comorbidity with other conditions can also lead to challenges in terms of diagnosis and can result in young people being described as 'complex' or perplexing.

Attention deficit hyperactivity disorder (ADHD) is a good example of this. Autism and ADHD are regarded as distinct and separate disorders in the DSM-5 (APA 2013) and, in previous versions of the DSM, autism was an exclusion criterion for ADHD, leading to the two disorders being treated separately for many years. More recent research has acknowledged that there appears to be considerable genetic, clinical and neuropsychological overlap between the two conditions (Rommelse *et al.* 2010, 2011), and they are now frequently diagnosed together.

A variety of studies have indicated that between 22 and 83 per cent of young autistic individuals will display some features of ADHD (Matson, Rieske and Williams 2013; Ronald *et al.* 2008) and between 30 and 65 per cent of young people with ADHD will display features of autism (Clark *et al.* 1999; Ronald *et al.* 2008). However, in terms of clinical assessment, this can lead to difficulties in differentiating the two conditions, particularly with regard to identifying the underlying autism which may be present, as both conditions can result in social communication and executive function difficulties. Episodes of 'challenging' behaviour are also observed, and this can, once again, lead to the child or young person being described as 'complex'.

Sokolova, Oerlemans and Rommelse (2017) outline the difficulties facing clinicians conducting assessments, as the inattentiveness and impulsivity that is typical in young people with ADHD frequently results in the child missing important social cues, displaying a tendency to interrupt and talk over others. In addition, a reduced ability to think ahead and foresee consequences can also lead to the child appearing to lack 'social imagination', which is also frequently seen in autistic children and young people.

In contrast many young people who receive a primary diagnosis of ADHD fail to have their underlying autism identified because they do not, at first glance, appear to have the need for repetition and routine typically associated with autism. However, having spoken with dual-diagnosed adults, it would appear that, for some at least, they are to all intents and purposes experiencing an internal battle between impulsive behaviour and a need for structure. Digby Tantam, a leading psychiatrist (Tantam 2012), described a group of individuals (mostly boys) who were both autistic and had ADHD as 'atypical'. These were young people who, at that time, did not fit the generally accepted picture of autism as they tended to have had disrupted educational experiences, had been labelled as 'naughty' or 'difficult' and were frequently excluded or expelled from school. Consequently, their difficulties were infrequently assessed or identified. In adolescence particularly, this often led to the young person becoming extremely vulnerable. It is not unusual for young people with this dual diagnosis to come into contact with the criminal justice system (CJS), where their underlying autism may continue to be missed. This issue will be covered in further detail in Chapter Seven.

In the DSM-IV (APA 1994), ADHD was included under the category of 'Attention Deficit and Disruptive Behavior Disorders', alongside ODD and conduct disorder. However, since the publication of the DSM-5, ADHD now appears under 'Neurodevelopmental Disorders', whereas ODD and conduct disorder now appear under the general heading of 'Disruptive/Impulse Control Disorders', alongside pyromania, kleptomania and 'Intermittent Explosive Disorder'.

Autism and ODD

Many autistic children are also diagnosed with ODD. The definition of what constitutes oppositional behaviour is one which has been the subject of much debate. The second edition of a book on the topic, published in 2017 (Matthys and Lochman 2017), outlines the ethical and clinical concerns involved in labelling young people according to the level of emotional dysregulation they display and the level to which they engage in behaviour that is deemed 'antisocial', inasmuch as the extent to which they are reluctant to comply with the requests of others and have a tendency towards violence. The formal definition of ODD describes a persistent pattern that includes anger, irritability and vindictive behaviour that has lasted at least six months and does not involve siblings.

According to one study (Lavigne *et al.* 2015), cited by Matthys and Lochman (2017), ODD can be conceptualised as having two dimensions – behavioural (argumentative) defiant behaviour and affective (anger/irritable mood), whereas conduct disorder as a diagnosis suggests that the young person has significantly violated societal norms in terms of either aggression towards people or animals, destruction of property, deceitfulness/theft and failing to follow rules. Many of these young people will also display higher levels of callous-unemotional traits, characterised by a lack of guilt or remorse and a lack of concern for the feelings of others (for a review see Frick *et al.* 2014).

A developmental psychopathology perspective on both of these 'disorders' examines the interaction between 'child factors' and 'context and experiential factors'. What this means, in reality, is that links are often made between children and young people presenting with these types of behaviour and 'hostile and inconsistent' parenting. In addition, as further pointed out in Matthys and Lochman (2017), disruptive behaviour and lack of compliance have been strongly linked to what they refer to as 'maternal guidance'. They also point to a positive correlation between sound maternal attachment and fewer negative behaviours.

PDA and autism

This then leads on to the debate around PDA, which perhaps contributes more to the discussion around complex and perplexing presentations than any other behavioural profile. It remains controversial, and while some areas within the United Kingdom have now developed dedicated pathways to support young people and their families, there are also a significant number of areas who fail to recognise that it exists. Because so many of the behavioural features are similar to those displayed by young people with other difficulties such as ODD, an assumption may be made that there must be parenting difficulties or attachment problems. However, my extensive clinical experience in this area has demonstrated that the majority of children and young people presenting with this type of difficulty come from supportive families who often have other children, brought up in exactly the same environment, who do not present with the same level of 'challenging' behaviour. In addition, rather than there being a problem with the parent-child attachment, children with the PDA profile are often almost over-attached to their parents (more commonly the mother).

Much of the debate around what the PDA profile is, and where it fits diagnostically, has come about as a result of the slowly developing understanding of the breadth and depth of what is now referred to as the autistic spectrum.

PDA (or pathological demand avoidance) was first discussed in the 1980s by child psychologist Elizabeth Newson (Newson 1983), initially when she was assessing children for autism. At that time, diagnosis of autism was made using DSM-III (APA 1980) criteria. Autism and related disorders were grouped under the heading of 'Pervasive Developmental Disorders' (PDD) and an 'atypical' category was also included. Elizabeth Newson initially argued that the group of children she assessed fitted some, but not all, of the criteria for autism (as they were understood at the time). She initially felt that PDA should be viewed as a separate (but related) condition, or 'syndrome', within the broader category of 'Pervasive Developmental Disorders'.

Over the years, and following the publication of the DSM-5, the diagnostic criteria for autism spectrum disorder has changed to reflect the growing understanding of the complex nature of autism, and it is likely that many of her original cohort of children would today meet the diagnostic criteria for autism.

In recent years in the United Kingdom, PDA has become more widely acknowledged as a behaviour profile seen in some autistic children (O'Nions *et al.* 2014). Many parents report experiencing a 'lightbulb' moment when they read about it for the first time and a strong sense of recognition of the profile. A paper by Green *et al.* (2018) highlighted the challenges faced by clinicians when families arrive for assessment who feel that this behaviour profile fits their child, particularly as there are still no clear and universally agreed criteria for it. Green *et al.* concluded that there was insufficient evidence to support classifying PDA as a separate profile, although they did acknowledge that there is a group of children who do present with extreme demand avoidance behaviour.

Over the past 20 years, I have been involved in the assessment and diagnosis of close to two thousand children. As a clinician, I have seen clear evidence of similarities in the way children behave and react to certain situations and a very definite pattern. All the children I have assessed have met criteria for autism first, although I am aware that some people feel that the PDA profile can exist in non-autistic people.

The key characteristics of the PDA profile, as initially described by Elizabeth Newson, are an obsessive resistance to everyday demands and requests; use of socially manipulative or outrageous behaviour to avoid demands; sudden changes in mood apparently associated with a need to control; and 'surface' sociability, reflected in social peculiarity, difficulties with peers and a lack of social constraint (Newson, LeMarechal and David 2003).

It is important, though, to acknowledge that not every child who resists demands or displays what can be seen as 'challenging' behaviour fits the PDA profile. All children are likely to display this type of behaviour at some point, indeed most adults do at times! Some children and young people resist particular activities that they find difficult or do not like.

Crucially though, the demand avoidance seen in children with the PDA profile (and, more importantly, by the young people themselves) is reported as pervasive and across all contexts. It can involve activities that they enjoy or even the most basic activities of eating and drinking. Many describe an 'invisible barrier' that stops them from engaging. In some, this leads to a need to control every aspect of their environment, including siblings and parents, making family life almost impossible. Parents often report that they are 'walking on eggshells', trying to avoid conflict and 'meltdowns'. 'Meltdowns', when they do occur, can be dramatic and last for many hours, with the young person appearing out of control and extremely distressed.

Key features of the PDA profile are now thought to be (Eaton and Weaver 2020):

- superficial/surface sociability – this usually means that the young person has the ability to 'mask' and may not initially be identified as having social difficulties. This can involve behaviour that is copied or mimicked from peers, or even TV and YouTube channels. It is not unusual for the young person to be able to 'hold it together' outside of the family home
- obsessively resists/avoids ordinary demands – as described above, the type of demand avoidance seen in young people with the PDA profile goes beyond simple avoidance of tasks that are unpleasant or difficult
- blaming other people – it can be difficult for some young people with the PDA profile to acknowledge their own part in situations that have gone wrong
- socially shocking or outrageous behaviour – this may involve public 'meltdowns' or deliberately breaking something. There is often less concern in these moments about whether peers witness this than might be the case in other children or young people
- manipulation (or negotiating excessively) – parents often report that young people with this profile will always try to

work towards a better 'deal' when asked to do something. This can involve relentless questioning or bargaining with parents that, once again, can go on for hours (or even days)

- communication through dolls/toys – some children with this profile will either talk through a doll or toy or respond better when parents use a doll or toy to make a request on their behalf
- dominating or bossy towards peers – many children with this profile, although socially motivated at a level, can struggle to compromise and play collaboratively with peers. They may insist upon the game being played 'their way' and may lose friends as a result
- strong fascination towards particular people – very often this can involve an over-attachment to one parent, often the mother, but it can also extend towards friends or celebrities
- rapid inexplicable changes in mood – this is often a key feature noted by parents of young people with the PDA profile and, indeed, the young people themselves. They often appear to become angry and upset very quickly, often with no apparent trigger
- comfortable in role play and fantasy – many children with the PDA profile display more imaginative play than other autistic children. They may totally 'get into a role' and insist that they are this character or enjoy rich fantasy play
- elaborate excuses – many young people with this profile devise elaborate and often inventive reasons why they are unable to do something, often claiming that 'their legs don't work', or they can't comply because 'they are a cat and a cat does not have hands'
- sabotaging (things that the child really wanted to do) – this is also a common feature of the PDA profile: sometimes a child or young person will appear to spoil or sabotage an activity they know, and parents know, they usually enjoy
- occasional extreme aggression or alternatively a complete 'shutdown' – this seems to result from a loss of control

- ineffectiveness of traditional reward and consequence-based parenting strategies – parents often report having attended parenting courses, only to find that the strategies suggested make their home situation worse.

Underpinning these difficulties are, in my clinical experience, the core autistic difficulties, even if they present in a less than 'typical' way. An example of this can be seen below where it is demonstrated how a child with the PDA profile might fit the DSM-5 criteria for autism. It is worth noting that (as initially identified by Elizabeth Newson) the gender distribution is close to 1:1 male to female, with many people initially wondering whether the PDA profile might represent a more 'female' presentation of autism. More recently, it is becoming more widely accepted that the old 'gendered' versions of autism may not be reflected in binary gendered presentations:

How the child with a PDA profile may fit the DSM-5 criteria

Social communication and interaction:

- *Social Emotional Reciprocity:* The child with the PDA profile may present with difficulties in engaging in back-and-forth conversations: there is often a reduced sharing of interests and emotions within social interactions.
- Non-verbal communication: Although the child may superficially appear to make good eye contact, this can often be poorly regulated and not integrated with facial expression and gestures. Some gestures may appear exaggerated. The child may misinterpret tone of voice and assume that someone is angry with them when they are not.
- Developing, maintaining and understanding relationships: The child is often reported to have 'friends'. It is not altogether clear that these are truly reciprocal relationships. The child may endeavour to control all interactions, and relationships can become intense and overwhelming at times.

Restricted repetitive patterns of behaviours, activities or interests (at least two of the following should be present for a diagnosis to be made):

- Stereotyped or repetitive behaviours. Few stereotyped and repetitive behaviours are seen in this group of young people.
- Insistence on sameness and routine. Children can be very specific about how they want things done, and can appear quite controlling. They are often reported as being 'on their own agenda'. They may be less willing, or able, to follow someone else's agenda.
- Highly restricted or fixated interests. Most children with this profile will present with strong interests. However, these can often be obsessions with people.
- Hyper or hypo reactivity to sensory input. Children will often have a number of sensory issues that impact upon their daily functioning.

The underlying driver for this type of presentation, apart from underlying autism, is thought to be anxiety, leading to the child or young person needing to have total control over their environment.

The whole picture described above sounds incredibly negative. However, without exception, parents of these young people report that when they are calm, the young person can be loving and caring and often feels bad after a 'meltdown' or disagreement, all of which do not fit the picture of a child diagnosed with ODD or conduct disorder.

Perhaps the most important message that came across loud and clear to us as clinicians working in this area was that traditional parenting techniques do not tend to work with children with the PDA profile, whereas behavioural techniques, such as rewards and consequences, tend to be more effective with young people who are labelled as having ODD or conduct disorder. This is often where the problems start when parents seek support from professionals. If it is assumed that a child's 'behaviour' is due to poor parental boundaries or insecure attachment to a primary caregiver, the advice given is often that parents should attend a parenting course. Parenting courses tend to focus upon providing the child with clear boundaries and having clear 'consequences' for behaviour that is deemed to be unacceptable. Very often, trying to implement these strategies ends up making the situation for parents and young people even more challenging. Anxiety levels on both sides rise and further difficulties appear, sometimes to the point that the child's mental health deteriorates or the situation at home becomes untenable.

So, what should parents do? Whilst it is clear that these children and young people are anxious and distressed, and the idea of consequences and 'punishment' does not feel right, it is clearly not appropriate or practical to have no boundaries. It is also important to manage the needs of the family and other children alongside supporting a young person who is clearly struggling.

The message that my team and I frequently give to parents is to 'pick your battles'. Some aspects of life are non-negotiable and must happen. However, other things, such as insisting upon homework being completed, taking a shower every day, or eating meals with the family, for example, may need to be put to one side, in order to focus on things that are potentially damaging or likely to cause significant harm.

Finally, as this is still a relatively new and contentious description, it can be difficult to find physicians or psychologists who either know about the PDA profile or accept that it is a 'thing'. Parents often have to research and explore many different avenues to try to get support and help and sometimes seek multiple assessments from different professionals. Unfortunately, this can be seen as a negative, and some parents have even found themselves accused of 'making up' or exaggerating their child's difficulties, especially if these are not observed outside of the home. It is to be hoped that, going forward, clinicians become more aware of 'perplexing and complex' presentations such as the PDA profile and that the evidence base continues to grow as more people become aware of it.

The impact of adverse childhood events

It is also well documented that children and young people who have experienced significant adverse childhood events or known developmental trauma can also present a diagnostic dilemma for assessing clinicians. Frequently, adopted or fostered children are taken for assessment because adoptive parents or carers suspect they may be autistic. Once again, these children are often described as 'complex' or 'challenging'. Little is often known with any degree of accuracy about the developmental history of their birth parents. Many will themselves have experienced disruptive or traumatic childhoods, which raises the issue of intergenerational trauma. In some cases, it is known that one or both birth parents were autistic or had other neurodevelopmental challenges, but this is by no means always clear.

The impact of adverse childhood events can be significant and far reaching. Children often present at paediatric and child and adolescent services with a range of complex behavioural difficulties, which frequently results in a variety of diagnoses.

Traditionally, individuals who experienced 'trauma' were diagnosed with post-traumatic stress disorder (PTSD). This was often following an isolated incident, such as witnessing an accident or an act of war, serious injury, or a physical or sexual assault (Davidson *et al.* 1991). Whilst in the early days of trauma research the focus was primarily on those individuals who developed disabling psychological, physiological and somatic symptoms upon their return from war zones, it was later found that the same features were observed in individuals within the community who had been exposed to distressing events. It also became clear that repeated or chronic stress in childhood can produce similar reactions.

When the DSM-IV was under development, the American Psychiatric Association (APA) organised a study, or 'field trial', to examine the impact of chronic 'developmental' trauma which was, at this time, labelled as 'disorders of extreme stress, not otherwise specified' (DESNOS). Various symptoms were examined, including changes in the ability to modulate emotions and 'alterations' in relationships with others. This was not listed as a separate diagnosis but was included under the umbrella label of PTSD. In later years more evidence has emerged regarding both the developmental and neurobiological consequences of early exposure to traumatic events. Researchers focused upon John Bowlby's (1988) work which highlighted the potential negative impact of parents who were not able to respond to a child in a timely way. The theory was that if parents were dealing with their own trauma and loss, they would be unable to be available as a source of safety and 'emotional containment' for their own children. This was then hypothesised to lead to the child exhibiting distress behaviour and to mistrust the safety of the world around them.

Bessel Van der Kolk (Van der Kolk *et al.* 2009) proposed a new diagnostic classification of developmental trauma prior to the publication of the DSM-5. However, it was not included. Although the proposed criteria for developmental trauma disorder (DTD) do not specifically mention attachment, the role of appropriate and protective early care was clearly acknowledged.

In a study by Tarren-Sweeney (2013), it was found that a third of 4–11-year-olds in care demonstrated some level of psychopathology, with a further 20 per cent displaying 'complex difficulties' which were difficult to conceptualise. These children were deemed to be up to four times more likely to develop a personality disorder than their non-traumatised peers.

In the original developmental trauma model, Van der Kolk (2005) theorised that later positive attachment experiences could mediate the impact of the earlier trauma and lead to better outcomes. However, the failure to include developmental trauma within the diagnostic manuals leaves clinicians and others working with these children and young people with an ongoing challenge of how to describe the difficulties they and their families often face. Van der Kolk further noted that many children who have experienced early trauma fall through the diagnostic net and either fail to receive a diagnosis or are given an incorrect diagnosis. Worse still, many are dismissed as 'too complex' for existing services. Few are offered a comprehensive assessment for autism.

This then leads on to consideration of the potential impact of in-utero drug or alcohol exposure. The impact of alcohol on the developing foetus is now well documented. Long-term neurobiological consequences of drinking alcohol during pregnancy include global and specific cognitive deficits, behavioural problems and neurodevelopmental delay. The effects are more marked when higher levels of alcohol are consumed. However, there are significant challenges about accurate reporting of alcohol consumption and what actually constitutes 'heavy drinking'.

The potential impact of recreational drugs on both short- and long-term neurodevelopment remains mixed and somewhat unclear. Despite babies being born to drug-addicted mothers suffering from neonatal withdrawal symptoms, the resulting cognitive and behavioural difficulties often observed in these children can be difficult to interpret, as many go on to experience adverse postnatal environments, which are believed to be mediated if the child is subsequently removed from that environment.

For clinicians attempting to distinguish between foetal alcohol syndrome (FAS) and autism, the paper by Bishop, Gahagan and Lord (2007) noted that both FAS and autism are characterised by difficulties with social interaction. Children with FAS very often display features that look similar to autism, for example cognitive delay, sensory sensitivities, deficits in executive function and poor adaptive functioning skills. Their social difficulties often include challenges in accurately perceiving social cues and problems in exercising good judgement in social interactions, which can interfere with friendships and peer relationships. However, Bishop *et al.* found that autistic children were likely to display a greater range of difficulties in social interaction in addition to restrictive interests and rigid thinking. Their most significant finding was that autistic children displayed significantly greater reduced frequency when evaluating the amount of attempts they made to initiate social interaction or respond to others' attempts to engage them.

Personality disorders

Finally in this chapter, we need to briefly discuss the issue of personality 'disorders'. For the past 40 years, intensive study has taken place regarding the diagnostic profile, longitudinal course, genetics and the neurobiological profile of what is referred to as 'emotionally unstable personality disorder'. It seems important to include this information, if only to understand why so many autistic people are labelled as having EUPD and why this is also often included as an additional (or comorbid) diagnosis.

The traditional approach taken in terms of diagnosis is that a person needs to display five out of nine of the following 'behaviours':

1. Fear of abandonment
2. Relational instability

3. Issues around identity
4. Impulsivity
5. Suicidal behaviour
6. Affective instability
7. Feelings of chronic emptiness
8. Intense anger
9. Transient paranoia

It is not difficult to imagine how many autistic people could potentially meet these criteria, particularly with regard to issues around identity, impulsivity and affective instability.

However, it is also extremely likely that, in many autistic people, these issues have only arisen because of a lack of understanding of their autism and inappropriate support being offered to them when they first began to show signs of distress.

Complications can arise though, when one considers the reasons why other individuals may develop behaviour that, on the surface, looks very similar. Many people who have experienced early trauma, adverse childhood experiences or disruption to their attachment to their primary caregivers will also display the type of behaviour that has been deemed to indicate the presence of a personality disorder.

So for the person whose 'behaviour' has resulted from the experiences they had as an undiagnosed, or misunderstood, autistic individual, it can continue to be difficult to secure the right kind of treatment and support, particularly as many services specialise in either personality disorders, or autism and learning disability. Few manage to combine both.

This lack of awareness and understanding can further add to the challenges experienced by autistic individuals who are also given a diagnosis of EUPD, especially if they are unfortunate enough to need an inpatient admission. A paper by Weight and Kendal (2013) outlines some of the negative perceptions around EUPD and the impact that this can have upon patient care.

EUPD is not always perceived as a 'genuine' mental illness, due to an assumption that it has no clear biological, or causal, pathway (Kendell 2002). Individuals diagnosed with EUPD are around 50 times more likely to die from suicide than the general population, and there appears to be a continuing stigma associated with being diagnosed (Leichsenring *et al.* 2011). According to the Weight and Kendal (2013) paper, this appears to be further compounded by the negative attitudes of some health care professionals. Service users often felt 'blamed' for their diagnosis and were made to feel that it was somehow their fault. They are also often perceived as 'manipulative' and in control of both their emotions and their reactions. Mental health nurses were reported as keeping a greater distance on inpatient wards from patients diagnosed with EUPD and were more likely to withdraw and present as less empathetic when the individual displayed 'challenging behaviour' or self-harm (Fraser and Gallop 1993). Negative behaviour is often perceived as deliberate (Forsyth 2007; Markham and Trower 2003).

Summary

To summarise, it can be seen from the examples in this chapter that there are a variety of ways in which children can be perceived as 'complex' or 'perplexing'. These also highlight the importance for clinicians of getting it right in terms of a diagnosis. Subsequent chapters include examples of what can go wrong if the right support is not put in place and the consequences when this does not happen.

CHAPTER TWO

Misdiagnosis and Missed Diagnoses in Women and Girls

This chapter will further address the issue of missed diagnosis, or misdiagnosis, in women and girls, including how individuals who are non-binary or present in an atypical manner are often missed in terms of an autism diagnosis.

There now exists a growing research literature that supports the gender differences in the way in which autism presents. However, considering this as a straightforward male/female dichotomy is somewhat misleading. In my clinical practice, my colleagues and I have frequently assessed children and young people who have been missed or misdiagnosed in terms of an autism diagnosis. We have seen girls who present as autistic in a more stereotypical 'male' way and an equal number of boys who present in what has come to be considered as a more 'female' way. This is without considering those who identify as transgender or non-binary. For these individuals, what can be perceived as a 'typical' presentation becomes further confused. The literature has, however, begun to reflect the issues I alluded to in my previous book – *A Guide to Mental Health Issues in Girls and Young Women on the Autism Spectrum* (Eaton 2017). This book was written between 2015 and 2017, and, in some ways, it is quite saddening that several years on there remain a considerable number of autistic people who remain undiagnosed, or misdiagnosed, simply because this new literature and thinking does not appear to be fully filtering through to clinicians who are responsible for making diagnoses.

In this book, I noted that many psychiatrists did not receive adequate (if any) training in autism. Certainly, this was the case for those who specialised in adult mental health. Thankfully, there now appears to be a growing awareness and understanding, certainly amongst new trainees entering the profession. This even extends into the area of perinatal mental health and autistic mothers, which is a huge step forward. However, the fact remains that there are still professionals, often acting as 'responsible clinicians' in inpatient and outpatient units, who appear not to appreciate the huge impact that being un- or mis-diagnosed can have on an autistic person.

It is now acknowledged that there are a number of different autistic phenotypes, psychiatric comorbidities and significant levels of 'masking' or camouflaging that can make the diagnostic process more challenging.

It may help to clarify how these challenges have emerged. Autism was first 'identified' in the 1940s by Leo Kanner and Hans Asperger respectively (Asperger 1944; Kanner 1943). In their initial studies few girls were included, and those who were tended to have intellectual disability and most closely fitted the narrow understanding of autism at that time, in that they often had little or no speech, presented as socially detached, and displayed stereotyped and repetitive movements. Over the years that followed, gender rates of three to four boys for every one girl diagnosed were repeatedly cited (e.g. Fombonne 2009), clearly based upon this early understanding. Some studies only examined the presentation of males.

A study by Kreiser and White (2014) noted that generally autistic females tend to engage in more sophisticated pretend play from an early age, use more emotionally expressive language and have a greater desire to interact socially compared to their male counterparts. In addition, they noted that autistic females tend to have fewer restrictive or obsessive interests compared to autistic males and that the interests they do have may be connected to celebrities or animals. The study also noted a higher-than-expected level of eating disorders amongst autistic females and a tendency towards perfectionism. Green *et al.* (2019) also noted that it has only been fairly recently that any information about a possible female phenotype for autism has started to emerge. However, as stated in the previous chapter, these differences can be subtle and not that far removed from what are perceived as neurotypical interests. As a result, they can be difficult to spot in a standard autism diagnostic assessment.

Using the DSM-5 criteria for autism in assessing girls

The outline below, although by no means exhaustive, demonstrates how, by using the DSM-5 criteria for autism, it is possible to provide a template for assessing girls.

Social Communication and Interaction

Social Emotional Reciprocity

Autistic girls tend to be somewhat more skilled at engaging in to and fro conversation. They are likely to have observed and/or mimicked their peers. However, there is likely to be a tendency for girls to have poor pragmatic (social use of) language skills. This may mean they interrupt or fail to realise that they are speaking too much, or too fast. They may also not realise when their listener has lost interest or wishes to move onto a different topic. They are also likely to misunderstand or misinterpret what has been said to them. This is often the area which causes the most anxiety and concern – negotiating complex relationships – as people do not always say what they mean, which can be challenging. Autistic adult females often report developing 'scripts' and learning 'how to do' small talk. They also report high levels of anxiety about getting social interaction 'wrong' and of being judged by their peers, often replaying conversations repeatedly in their head to work out whether they have said, or done, something wrong.

Non-Verbal Communication

This is perhaps the one area which provides the greatest challenge when assessing and diagnosing girls and women. Autistic girls become skilled at observing and copying their peers and will almost always be seen to use gestures and facial expressions. They may also appear outwardly more comfortable making and maintaining eye contact. However, when speaking to autistic women, they will often say how stressful and uncomfortable this actually is. Also, if watched carefully, it is possible to pick up subtle difficulties with non-verbal communication; gestures may be over-exaggerated and slightly 'off' in terms of timing. For many British girls, a slight trace of an American accent is often picked up, or they may use phrases that sound scripted or culturally inappropriate. This is because many admit to watching American TV programmes or YouTube videos to try to 'learn' the rules of social interaction.

Developing, Maintaining and Understanding Relationships

Many autistic girls, despite being socially motivated, struggle to make, and more importantly maintain, peer relationships. Some may appear over-controlling, operating better in a dyad with one other peer. Groups of three or more can be difficult, or even impossible, to negotiate. Autistic girls and adult women can find it hard to repair or put relationships back on track after any conflict. Parents of autistic girls report that they have to work hard to 'scaffold' their daughters' relationships. Many go on to be vulnerable in terms of relationships, particularly during the teenage years, often becoming at risk of being bullied or taken advantage of. A number find that they struggle with adult romantic relationships and find themselves embroiled in coercive or abusive relationships. Again, there is often a sense of almost, but not quite, getting things right.

Restrictive Repetitive Patterns of Behaviour, Activities, or Interests

This is often the area where clinicians struggle to see how autistic girls meet the diagnostic criteria.

Stereotyped and Repetitive Behaviours

These tend to be observed less frequently in girls, not necessarily because they engage in them any less, but more often because their desire to fit in means they will 'mask' or try to cover up any repetitive movements or 'stims'. Somewhat like the tics observed in Tourette's Syndrome, these 'stims' are only carried out in private when the young person is alone.

Insistence on Sameness and Routine

The majority of autistic girls will easily fulfil this criterion, although a need for routine and sameness and concerns about transitions can often be attributed solely to anxiety.

Highly Restricted or Fixated Interests

These tend to be far less obvious in autistic girls. Many of the interests they pursue are similar to, or copied from, their neurotypical peers. Pop groups, celebrities and animals do tend to be popular, as does Japanese anime. Dressing up or 'cosplay' are also favourite choices.

It has been observed that, generally, the play of autistic girls is more sophisticated than that of autistic boys. However, it is important to explore the nature of this play a little more. Although, superficially, it might look very good, there will often be a great deal of 'setting up' of scenes or replaying scenes from school. Playing with peers can also present challenges as it can be difficult for the autistic girl to continue with a game if it veers away from the 'script' that she had in her head.

Hypo- or Hyper-reactivity to Sensory Input

This is another area that is often overlooked in autistic girls, as once again, many girls try hard to camouflage or mask their challenges. However, this frequently leads to stress, sensory overload, 'meltdown' and ultimately burnout.

Effects of diagnosis on women

Went (2016) carried out a qualitative analysis of women's experiences relating to a diagnosis of autism, entitled 'I didn't fit the stereotype of autism'. She reported a number of 'themes', the first of which was 'Feeling Different', with many women identifying that from a very early age they knew they were 'different' to the rest of the world. A second theme was 'Hiding Self' where women reported spending their entire lives carefully observing how neurotypical people behave so they could 'act like them and not stand out from the crowd like a weirdo' (Went 2016, p.68). 'Being Misunderstood' was also a commonly reported theme which resulted in a significant impact upon self-esteem and anxiety levels. The study then outlined how often a chance remark encouraged them to start to research autism and how, frequently, this led to a sense of relief. A final theme that emerged related to the ongoing struggle to obtain a formal diagnosis and an observation about the lack of measures to diagnose adults and even fewer for adult females.

It was also noted that, even after a formal diagnosis, many women were not believed when they disclosed this to health professionals. Often their motivation for seeking a diagnosis was questioned, and some were told that they were functioning 'too well' to be autistic and had their diagnoses completely refuted or replaced with something else (usually EUPD, bi-polar affective disorder or psychosis).

As a result of being misunderstood, or not believed, the women in the Went (2016) study reported a high number of comorbid mental health conditions, including anxiety, panic disorders and phobias. Others reported depression, fear, anger, loneliness and shame.

Autism and gender dysphoria

It is also important at this juncture to briefly discuss the issue of co-occurring autism and gender dysphoria. It would be wrong to discuss the 'male' and 'female' presentations of autism without acknowledging that for many this binary distinction is not helpful.

Turban and van Schalkwyk (2018) discussed seven out of 19 available studies reporting the over-occurrence of autism/autistic 'traits' in gender dysphoric/diverse individuals and felt that it was difficult to make an unequivocal link (partly because not all participants in these studies were formally diagnosed). However, this was countered by Strang *et al.* (2018a) who outlined seven studies that specifically reported autism diagnoses amongst gender diverse individuals. These seven studies all showed a significantly greater occurrence of clinically confirmed autism diagnoses in those who identified as gender diverse. Autism diagnoses were reported to be between 4.1 and 17.5 times more common than in the general population. All the authors who contributed to the Strang *et al.* (2018a) study were either clinicians or researchers in the area of autistic transgender identity and were keen to stress the issues that this can raise in terms of gender needs, gender exploration and gender 'affirmation' (previously known as gender transition).

The whole issue of gender dysphoria in autism has implications in terms of diagnosis and, in particular, misdiagnosis. There has been a growing interest in recent years in both gender dysphoria and sexuality, so it is challenging to unpick whether this apparent rise in the number of autistic individuals who identify as gender dysphoric simply reflects a greater tolerance and awareness of the issue in society.

Gender dysphoria as described in the DSM-5 refers to the distress experienced by those who feel their assigned gender does not reflect their preferred gender. Gender dysphoria is, by definition, categorical, whilst gender nonconformity (GNC) is a more dimensional construct and includes those individuals who are not necessarily seeking gender reassignment treatment.

Individuals who are assigned male at birth and who identify as female are described as AMAB, whereas females who identify as males are described as AFAB. Historically gender dysphoria was more commonly reported in those assigned male at birth. However, for adolescents in particular, the sex ratio has shifted to include more females at birth. Heylens *et al.* (2018) reported an over-representation of autistic traits and autism in both AMAB and AFAB individuals. In terms of assessment, they are recommending a longer assessment period for those with gender dysphoria and autism as they suggest that gender dysphoria-related symptoms could be mistaken for autism and vice versa.

Strang *et al.* (2018a) discuss the significant diagnostic challenges for clinicians when assessing autistic adolescents with gender dysphoria/gender nonconformity. They report that there were no guidelines for this prior to their study, which aimed to develop initial clinical guidelines for assessment. Strang *et al.* stress the importance of ensuring joined-up and collaborative clinical assessment that includes experts from both areas. They also suggest that all adolescents presenting at gender identity clinics should be screened for autism.

As stated previously in this chapter, many of the assessment tools for autism tend to favour the predominant 'male' stereotype and can be less effective at identifying those who do not conform to gender stereotypes.

The impact on mental health

The second part of the Went (2016) study explored (using a Grounded Theory approach) the impact of mis- or no diagnosis on mental health. She reported that in general women receive their autism diagnosis later than men (Geurts and Jansen 2012) and that the resulting (or prior) lack of both professional and self-understanding can lead to the development of mental health issues. This, in turn, can lead to the person's presentation being perceived as more 'complex' (Ghazziuddin 2005).

In contrast, the experience of being given a diagnosis was cited as 'transformational'. One woman wrote: 'I was diagnosed with ASD [autism spectrum disorder] earlier this year and it has literally been a lifesaver for me. Everything in my life is improving since the diagnosis and I feel I am getting a second chance to live by having this new understanding' (Went 2016, p.68).

However, some women continued to report feelings of anxiety, loneliness and depression and of struggling to come to terms with past events. Most found that medication or therapy that did not address how the core experience of having been misdiagnosed or undiagnosed autistic had impacted upon their mental health. It was also reported that the 'wrong' type of therapy had offered only a temporary solution to their difficulties. Many reported that they had struggled to come to terms with how things might have been different for them had they been diagnosed earlier. Sadly, many of them also noted that they continued to feel the need to 'mask' or camouflage their true selves.

It would appear that, in terms of therapeutic support post-diagnosis, what is most important is the practitioner's understanding of autism.

From a clinical perspective, what appears to be most helpful is for the practitioner first and foremost to have familiarised themselves with the way that many females (and transgender and non-binary persons) present as autistic. Diagnostic services are, and are likely to continue to be, overloaded and stretched in terms of capacity. Given that this is a factor that is unlikely to be quickly or easily resolved, it is helpful to consider the validity of self-identification and self-diagnosis. There is a growing amount of easily accessible information about females and autism. If an individual reads this and strongly feels that the description resonates with their own experiences, surely it would make sense for therapists and mental health practitioners to acknowledge this when offering therapy and support.

The type of therapy that may prove helpful for autistic females can include adapted cognitive behavioural therapy (CBT). However, this would need to take into account the challenges that some autistic persons have with interpreting the physiological emotional signals and the rigid thinking style that can impact upon the ability to 'challenge' a negative thought. Dialectical behaviour therapy (DBT) skills that include mindfulness, interpersonal effectiveness, distress tolerance and emotion regulation can also be helpful. However, individual sessions tend to work better than group sessions.

Acceptance and commitment therapy (ACT) can help individuals to identify and clarify their own personal values and goals whilst at the same time accepting and embracing their differences. Finally, some individuals may benefit from focused trauma work, such as eye movement desensitisation and reprocessing (EMDR).

Missed and misdiagnosis in motherhood

One final area where autistic women often go undiagnosed and misunderstood is when they become mothers. In recent years in the United Kingdom, specialist perinatal mother and baby wards have been set up in some hospitals across the country. As was the case with inpatient services, it has quickly become clear that many of the women suffering from postnatal psychosis are, in fact, undiagnosed autistic. A study by Pohl *et al.* (2020), which was the first of its kind, examined the key issues for autistic mothers in the perinatal period.

Pohl *et al.* make the point that due to missed or misdiagnosis many autistic mothers may have spent their whole lives not understanding their neurodiversity. So, when thinking about emotional dysregulation and 'challenging' or 'difficult' behaviour, it is important to understand where this has come from. They found that many autistic women experience a deep-seated fear of rejection or getting things wrong. Many of these fears can be amplified when they become new mothers. A number of mother and baby units have been set up across the UK recently to support mothers experiencing postnatal psychosis.

As part of putting together some training for perinatal psychiatrists, I interviewed autistic mothers and below are the findings combined with those from the Pohl *et al.* study, which outline areas where they experienced difficulties, and the ways in which they would like to be supported and, more importantly, where they may be misunderstood and perceived as 'complex' or 'challenging'.

The Pohl *et al.* study explored autistic mothers' experiences of the peri- and post-natal period and included:

- Pregnancy
- Childbirth
- The postpartum period
- Self-perceptions of parenting
- Identified strengths and weaknesses
- Mental health difficulties
- The social experience of motherhood

During pregnancy and childbirth, one of the key areas mentioned were sensory issues, both hyper- and hyposensitivity to aspects of pregnancy and birth such as morning sickness, feeling the baby's movements and reporting of contractions and labour pain. In the postpartum period, issues around the sensory experience of breastfeeding were also mentioned.

Many of the women felt unable to mention these aspects to professionals treating them and (if they were diagnosed) they were often reluctant to disclose this due to fear of being stigmatised as a 'bad mother' as a result of misconceptions around their parenting ability. This report highlights the need for the improved recognition of autism in new mothers and a potential need to develop specific tools to evaluate postnatal depression in autistic women, in order to minimise the risk of their challenges becoming more complex than they need to. This issue is discussed more fully in the next chapter, which is a personal perspective written by an autistic mother.

CHAPTER THREE

A Personal Account by an Autistic Mother

HADASSAH

This chapter is a personal account by an autistic mother who tells her story of how being autistic was misinterpreted by multiple professionals as postnatal depression and emotionally unstable personality disorder (EUPD) after the birth of her daughter. Hadassah[1] highlights the need for better understanding of autistic mothers, before, during and after the birth of their children. The words are her own and reflect her own personal journey.

In 2016, on an evening in June, I was sitting on my sofa, and I had the taste of metal in my mouth. At that point I knew that I was pregnant. The following day I took a test which confirmed that I was indeed pregnant.

I went into survival mode. A few years prior, I had lost a pregnancy. I quit smoking, started eating healthily and went for regular exercise each day. I wanted to give my pregnancy the best possible chance of going full term. I was convinced that I would not carry full term, and this fear made it very difficult for me to properly prepare. During my previous pregnancy I had bought many baby things. This was something

---

1   This is a pseudonym.

that I wasn't going to do again because the pain and shame I felt having to pack away the unused baby things, and sell them, was unbearable.

Months went by; I was the most stable I had ever been. Not having a period each month was such a relief. Since my periods started, I have never been able to cope with them; the emotional rollercoaster, having to contend with premenstrual tension and the physical sensation of losing blood each month impacted me massively as an autistic woman.

My approach to pregnancy and parenthood was logical. Retrospectively, my previous miscarriage had impacted me, although I didn't recognise that at the time because I have alexithymia. I find it difficult to recognise my emotions, let alone explain them. I did not know or understand how, or what, I was feeling, and because of lack of professional awareness around alexithymia, it was misunderstood that I did not want my baby. This was untrue. I so desperately wanted my baby; I simply responded to emotions in a different way.

Alexithymia

Alexithymia can occur in autistic and neurotypical people. Studies suggest 1 in 5 autistic people have alexithymia (De Berardis *et al.* 2017). There is not enough awareness around alexithymia and autism; many professionals including mental health professionals have never heard of the condition. This is very concerning because, as I have experienced, the absence of awareness and understanding can leave alexithymics vulnerable to being misunderstood, misdiagnosed, subjected to ineffective and/or unnecessary treatment, or being unfairly judged leading to devastating consequences. Research has highlighted the importance of alexithymia screening in everyday clinical practice (De Berardis *et al.* 2017). However, I am not convinced that this is happening, or that professionals truly understand the condition and how this presents in autistic people, particularly autistic females. Research suggests that people with alexithymia scarcely respond to both pharmacotherapy and psychotherapy (De Berardis *et al.* 2017), which bolsters the case for professional awareness. I have been subjected to treatment and therapy which was not effective. I accept that at the time I wasn't aware I had alexithymia nor were the professionals; however, the symptoms were there and, as a result of lack of awareness, the symptoms were misunderstood. Now that I am aware of it, I have a better understanding of the condition. However, despite this, it does appear that professionals do not understand the implications of the condition in relation to treatment and just perceive it as another unnecessary label. Within mental health and child protection it is paramount that professionals understand alexithymia, as without this understanding, alexithymic parents could be unfairly accused of detached or disassociated parenting. With the right understanding and support professionals will be able to support parents with identifying both their own emotions and the emotions of their children.

Pregnancy was a surreal experience; having something supposedly growing inside of you is rather an abstract concept. I struggled to come to terms with it right up until my daughter's birth, and even when my daughter was born via caesarean section, I still looked at her and was like – where on earth did you come from? Was I pregnant or have I just eaten an incredible amount of food? Autistic people struggle with abstract concepts; pregnancy is rather abstract, therefore it is likely that some autistic mothers will find pregnancy, particularly their first pregnancy, difficult to process.

My pregnancy experience was atypical, which led me to be heavily judged by others because I wasn't responding like a 'normal' mother. This judgement led me to believe that there was something wrong with me, and I asked for help. That is when social services got involved. Asking for their help, and allowing them into my life, was the worst mistake of my life. I trusted them and believed that they would help me adjust to becoming a parent. I was so wrong, but by the time I had realised, it was too late. They had already stolen my baby.

Social services involvement

When I met my first social worker, she seemed really kind and supportive, although, having said that, she was heavily focused on my misdiagnosis of EUPD. This has since been revoked, but unfortunately due to the gender bias within autism research largely focusing on the 'male' presentation of autism, autistic females have been consistently misunderstood, resulting in late or misdiagnosis. Many times, she put words into my mouth which were not true at the time. I queried these inaccuracies with her. However, months later, there was no acknowledgement of these challenges within her records.

My autism diagnosis was completely overlooked. Every behaviour was interpreted into a severe 'mental illness' mantra. When I challenged this with my community mental health nurse, instead of the social worker taking another look at my case, she decided that she had more qualifications than the mental health professionals. I was branded as the mother who lacked insight into her severe mental illness and someone who told different stories to different professionals.

In my third trimester I became all consumed by anxiety about becoming a mother. It was my first baby, and I couldn't imagine what it would be like or whether I would cope. The closest comparison I had was my training as a nursery nurse. I expressed my crippling anxieties about motherhood to social services, hoping that they would provide some reassurance and support. Unfortunately, I was repeatedly told that social services could not offer any support until after the birth. I was told to 'wait and see'. For me my anxiety became so overwhelming, I felt crippled and suffocated; this could have been reduced by simply, and practically, addressing my anxieties. There was a lack of understanding from social services and the midwifery team about the barriers autistic parents face in accessing antenatal classes. No alternative was considered; it was assumed that I simply didn't want to engage or become a mother.

What I feel needs to change is early support. I would like to see more awareness around anxiety, both prenatal and postnatal, in autistic mothers. Had a social worker taken the time to reassure me, work through my anxieties, offer practical support about how to make a bottle, talk through breastfeeding, changing a nappy, bathing a baby, or even holding a baby, this would have been so helpful and reduced my anxiety. Most of these activities I already knew how to do because of being a nursery nurse. However, at the time I was so crippled by anxiety and self-doubt I couldn't see a way forward.

I recognised that it would be difficult for me to have a natural birth. I find unpredictability very unsettling; I am better when I am prepared.

On the basis of my autism diagnosis, I requested a caesarean section, and a separate room if they had one available, due to my sensory processing difficulties. I do not regret this request; I made the right decision. The process was predictable and formulaic; I was able to plan and prepare. On the morning of my caesarean section, I was so calm. I cannot fault the section itself, and the hospital staff were very good at ensuring that I was given as much information as possible. However, the understanding stopped there. After the birth of my daughter, because my response was deemed 'atypical' and because I became mute (which I now understand was because of autism burnout), staff viewed me as a cold mother who didn't want or care for her baby and labelled me an 'attention seeker'. To make matters worse, social services would not allow me to go home with my baby. They 'gaslit' me into a voluntary admission to a mother and baby unit; I was told that if I wanted the best for my baby, I would accept the admission. The social worker filled me with fear, implying that it was a given that I would have postnatal depression and other mental health implications, so I needed to attend a mother and baby unit so that I could be kept under close supervision. The social worker convinced me and my family that it was inevitable that I would become severely mentally unwell, and that they urgently needed an interim care order. Not fully understanding what this was, we agreed that this was necessary.

While I was on the waiting list for a mother and baby unit bed to become available I had to remain in the maternity hospital. Hospitals are not autism friendly. They cause so many difficulties for me as an autistic person, and I find such places incredibly disabling. Poor understanding of this meant that mental health professionals, health professionals and social workers perceived the impact of the hospital environment as a deterioration in my misdiagnosed EUPD, resulting in further unnecessary judgement and treatment. Had my autism and the impact of the hospital environment been understood, I would have been afforded the opportunity to go home with my new baby, or reasonable adjustments would have been made so that I could function in an environment which was at odds with my autism.

Logomisia

After the birth of my daughter, it became apparent that I had an intense dislike for the word Mummy. At the time, logomisia (a term for a strong dislike for a particular word, or type of word, based upon its sound, usage or associations) was not considered; instead it was assumed that I had postnatal depression and was disassociated from becoming a mother. This was not true; I needed time to adjust. I was so overwhelmed, I was struggling to express how I was feeling. I had never been a mother before; it was a huge change. All my life I had only ever experienced being referred to by two names: Hadassah and my nickname. I struggled with the additional name, and to make matters worse the professionals working with me referred to me as 'Mummy' – which provoked an intense involuntary response of disgust. After the removal of my daughter, I spent time trying to understand why these words caused such distress, and that was when I became aware of logomisia. I started looking at other words that didn't cause so much distress and found the name Momma, which gave me an intense feeling of calmness and peace; from then on, I became a momma.

Reflecting back, I think one of the biggest problems in my case was the assumption by professionals prior to my daughter's birth that, because of the incorrect EUPD diagnosis I had at the time along with my autism diagnosis, I could not be a 'good enough' mother and that it was inevitable that I would have postnatal depression. This resulted in damaging assumptions and decisions being made without taking a deeper look at the evidence or the reasons behind the difficulties I was having.

Prosopagnosia (face blindness)

There is little awareness of face blindness, and this creates a further opportunity for my symptoms to be misunderstood by professionals. This is something that I experience; I have face blindness, and when I had my daughter superficial questioning and lack of awareness meant that my face blindness was misunderstood as postnatal depression and a detachment from my new role as a mother. Often face blindness goes unnoticed; many people adapt without even realising they have it. I had spent all my life recognising people by their hairstyles and smells. This helped me to understand why I would become distressed when people changed their hairstyle, and why I don't take photographs of people including myself because I struggle to recognise the people in the photographs.

Autism and breastfeeding

Before I was transferred to the mother and baby unit, I was shown how to breastfeed my baby. I wanted to breastfeed because I was aware of all the scientific benefits; what I was not prepared for was the impact it had on my autism. At the time there was a complete absence of understanding of the impact of breastfeeding on autistic mothers. All the approaches were for neurotypical mothers. An understanding of neurodiversity within breastfeeding support did not exist.

As I was breastfeeding it became apparent that I was struggling, but I didn't understand why. I felt agitated and overwhelmed. At times, I was extremely sensitive to touch, at other times I didn't feel anything and wouldn't recognise when I was hurting. The to and fro social interaction between my baby and me made me feel suffocated, and I withdrew from others. Many people told me that breastfeeding was enjoyable and facilitates a bond between mother and baby. Enjoyable is not a word that springs to mind when I look back on my breastfeeding experience. I would say it was more of a kaleidoscope of intense sensory input, along with waves of many overwhelming emotions and social suffocation. Breastfeeding as an autistic mother is complicated, but it is fair to say that a large number of autistic mothers want to breastfeed, despite the unique challenges we face.

I continued to force myself to breastfeed; I was determined to provide the most nutritious milk for my baby. I sought help and advice from professionals, but, unfortunately, this led to me being completely misunderstood. Once again, this led to snap judgements being made by professionals with devastating consequences. I was often told to give up breastfeeding when you would think they would have encouraged and supported me. My experience was that professionals were way too quick to recommend bottle feeding without any attempt to understand what I was experiencing as an autistic breastfeeding mother. If perinatal services understood that breastfeeding for autistic women can be a very different experience, they would be able to provide accessible and relatable support for autistic breastfeeding parents.

The absence of knowledge

A bed finally became available at a mother and baby unit which was hundreds of miles away from my home. However, this did not upset me too much as it was by the seaside, and I love the sea. This unit had a good awareness of autistic parenting. They were not in agreement with the diagnosis of EUPD and were very clear that the difficulties I was experiencing were autism related, not mental health related, and that I needed time to adjust. However, this was not what the social worker wanted to hear. The social worker became fixated on the EUPD misdiagnosis and was convinced that I was having a mental breakdown, which led to differences in opinion between the social worker and the mother and baby unit. This ultimately resulted in a working relationship breakdown between them and the social worker enforcing a medically unnecessary transfer to another unit. I was very clear that I did not want to transfer. Both the baby and I had settled in this unit. However, once again I was gaslighted and manipulated into agreeing to the transfer.

The second mother and baby unit had absolutely no understanding of autism. They viewed me through a mental health lens, and not at any point did they consider my autism, despite me raising concerns multiple times regarding the lack of reasonable adjustments they were making. The only time they considered my autism was when they wrote in my medical records: 'It's unrealistic to expect autistic parents to be able to parent long term.' Yet they had made no efforts to seek out specialised support or understand my autism. The second mother and baby unit assessed my parenting through a rigid, neurotypical lens. They used restrictive practices, lacked specialist expertise in autism, made limited attempts to seek specialist expertise and didn't afford me a specific sensory or environmental needs assessment. I felt judged. I felt like I was being set up to fail. I was in this unit for less than 10 days before social services applied for the removal of my baby. This information was withheld from me until it was too late. I was given less than 24 hours' notice that they were going to remove my baby. My legal team did me a disservice because they were focused on the diagnosis I had at the time. They didn't want to understand autism, and they had already decided that my case was hopeless. My legal team at the time of my daughter's removal were aware for seven days of the local authority's plan to remove, but they withheld this information. Had I been made aware of the plan I would have been able to provide evidence which could have prevented the unlawful removal of my daughter. The local authority told the court that my mental health had deteriorated and therefore my baby was at significant risk of serious harm. However, this was fabricated; all the medical evidence stated that my mental health was stable and keeping me in an inpatient setting was medically unnecessary. This was never put forward to the court at the time. The social worker decided I lacked capacity despite being told by medical professionals that I did have capacity and that a capacity assessment was unnecessary. This meant I had limited ability to fight or challenge the removal until the capacity assessment was completed. The local authority was granted permission to remove my daughter. My solicitor telephoned me to inform me of the news and I was told I had less than one hour to say goodbye to my seven-week-old baby. I have never been so distressed in my life; I was shaking and crying. I held my baby and breastfed her one last time. Nursing staff gathered all my baby's things, threw them into hospital bags and bin bags, and packed them up for the social worker to take to the foster carers. My friend was travelling to the mother and baby unit so that she could be with me when the social worker removed my baby. When my friend was 10 minutes away from the unit, she rang and begged them to wait for her to arrive, so I could have support. The social worker refused to wait. She took my baby and all her things; I was left with nothing apart from leaking breasts.

Once my baby had been taken, I was left on the unit waiting for my friend. I was extremely distressed. The nursing staff grabbed my belongings in front of me and shoved them into bags. They wanted me off the unit. I was followed everywhere; I wasn't even afforded the right to privacy in the bathroom.

I was treated like a sub-human by all involved. Prior to this experience, I was proud of being a British citizen because I thought I lived in an inclusive country. However, I am now ashamed of this country because of the hidden human rights violations this country subjects its citizens to. All this goes on out of sight, under the guise of child protection, the family courts and mental health units. The UK has worked to promote mental health awareness to end the stigma around mental health. It has also raised awareness around autism and various other hidden disabilities. However, hidden away, behind closed doors, the UK has a dirty secret: systemic poor treatment and human rights violations against patients within institutions meant to help and support. I have experienced and witnessed professionals employed by these institutions treat service users as sub-human; I have experienced being mocked by mental health professionals; I have witnessed it happening to other patients on the wards; and, despite complaining, our complaints are written off because we are the 'mentally ill' and they are the 'innocent, sane' professionals.

Autistic burnout misunderstood as postnatal depression

I was exhausted. In less than seven weeks, I had moved between three different hospitals. Each hospital had a different set of rules. Just as I was getting used to one set, I was moved to another hospital, only to find another set of rules, different staff and another environment.

Trying to keep up with all the different social aspects of the hospital environment was draining. On top of that, I had the added pressure to behave as a neurotypical mother. I was exhausted. All I had wanted was to be left alone and have time to adjust to my new baby. Shortly after the birth of my daughter I found myself physically unable to speak; I had absolutely no idea what was happening, neither did the professionals, and unfortunately, because of the EUPD misdiagnosis, professionals believed I was just trying to seek more attention. More attention was the last thing I wanted. I was exhausted, overloaded and overwhelmed. It took days for my speech to return; I ended up sleeping so much because of sheer exhaustion.

I believe that I was experiencing autism burnout, but this was never picked up; instead it was decided that I was experiencing postnatal depression. Autistic burnout is a likely possibility in autistic parents. If we break pregnancy and birth down and look at it through the autism lens, having a baby is an immensely socially demanding experience. In the run up to birth everyone, including people you don't know, asks you a million and one questions about the baby you are having. They ask you about baby names, what is the baby's gender, and they expect to see this super-happy mother-to-be. As an autistic mother with alexithymia, I wasn't super-happy or excited; I didn't really know how I felt, and I was fed up with people asking me, feeling this enormous expectation to be this perfect mother and respond in a way that was not natural for me. Many autistic mothers mask to try and fit in; however, over time as an autistic mother masking, I became more and more drained until I was so exhausted that I could no longer mask.

Autism burnout needs to be better understood by professionals. With the right understanding autistic mothers can recover from burnout. Unfortunately, I was not afforded this, and instead I was unnecessarily treated for postnatal depression. When the treatment did not work, instead of the medical staff taking a step back to consider autism-related burnout, they simply assumed that I was just not cut out to be a mother long term.

It is really important that all mother and baby units have specific autism parenthood training. Generic autism training is not enough when working with autistic parents and assessing their parenting inter-actions within an inpatient setting. I have had first-hand experience of how unhelpful a basic training in autism can be. From my experience, some staff who had received this training were less understanding than some staff with no training at all. Often the staff with basic autism training were too focused on the stereotypes and could not see past the deficit medical model and viewed me as a deficient parent from the outset.

Supervised contact

I agreed to go into an acute mental health unit to prove that my mental health was stable. However, during that time I became extremely distressed because of my baby being removed whilst a breastfeeding mother. I was not informed for over a week where my baby was. No words can describe how traumatic this was. I made many attempts to contact the social worker to find out where my baby was and when I could see her. It was quite clear that the social worker did not want to facilitate any bond between myself and my baby after her removal. Despite still trying to maintain breastfeeding, I was only allowed three hours a week supervised contact. Ultimately, because contact was so infrequent, I had no choice but to give up. I was eventually discharged from the acute mental health unit with no mental instability detected.

No reasonable adjustments were made to ensure contact was accessible. As an autistic person I find travelling rather difficult due to my crippling sensory sensitivities and the unpredictability of travelling. I am better at home, in my own environment. Despite this information being regularly disclosed to the local authority, they refused to make any reasonable adjustments for my autism. In fact, the social worker repeatedly told me that it was not about me; they were only there for the child. It was as if I was somehow asking for favourable treatment, rather than the reasonable adjustments that, by law, they should have endeavoured to make.

I had no choice but to travel miles away from my home to the supervised contact centre. The journey was often unpredictable, ranging from 30 minutes to over two hours depending on traffic and/or public transport. By the time I had arrived at the contact centre, I was in an extremely high state of distress. There was never a consistent room booked, and staff seemed to treat parents with contempt. Because of my travel-related difficulties and the hostility I experienced from staff, I eventually asked my advocate to come with me to support me.

The distress caused by the local authority refusing to make reasonable adjustments caused a relapse in a physical condition I have, and I ended up spending a week in hospital. It was at this point after months of refusal the local authority finally agreed to contact taking place at my home.

Supervised contact is not realistic. How can a parent demonstrate their full parenting capabilities when they are being watched, and judged, by supervisors who are not independent from the local authority? Most contact supervisors are registered with agencies; however, once they have been allocated contact to supervise, the agency takes no further responsibility for the worker. It could be suggested that there was a conflict of interest, and when looking at the quality and accuracy of my contact records, you would be forgiven in thinking so.

The local authority relied heavily on the supervised contact records. The contact supervisors would not allow me to have access to the written notes, and the local authority used every delaying tactic in the book to prevent me seeing them. This made me extremely suspicious, and, once I finally got my hands on the written contact records, my suspicions were confirmed. The contact records reflected the local authority's stance that I was emotionally cold towards my daughter and had poor parenting skills. I was so angry, I felt helpless; the local authority was actively trying to deceive the court. I had nowhere to turn. I complained to the local authority and the contact agency, but once again, I was treated with contempt and ignored.

I felt that I had no choice but to covertly video record my contact in a desperate attempt for the judge to see the truth. No parent should ever have to be put in this position. From my experience of child protection, it is so very easy for the current system to be manipulated by professionals: parents are helpless, and the courts are none the wiser. Article 6 in the Human Rights Act protects your right to a fair trial. From my experience child protection did not afford me the right to a fair trial, and I believe that many parents, including autistic parents, have not been afforded the right to a fair trial within the family courts. That said I do believe that some local authorities are better than others; however, regardless, this should not be happening. Children should not be being removed without good reason, and local authorities should not be able to provide anything other than a fully rounded picture to the courts particularly where removal of a child is being considered.

Going home to a house full of baby things

I remember going home alone to the house I had prepared for myself and my baby. Walking past the newly decorated nursery, I felt like my heart was being ripped out. I felt so alone. I felt like family, friends and even neighbours were secretly judging me. I felt so ashamed and so worthless. Trying to explain what had happened felt pointless because I didn't feel believed, and I knew others were judging, viewing me as this angry parent who couldn't accept she was a terrible mother. Consequently, I eventually hid away. The almost two years I was separated from my daughter were the most lonely and painful years of my life. The only way I managed to get through was by proving that the local authority had unlawfully removed my daughter and that is exactly what I did.

Operation Spud

I was on a mission; I knew that the local authority was hiding something. I knew that I had been set up to fail, and my daughter had been unlawfully removed from my care. I had to prove it. My word alone wasn't enough – that is when I launched Operation Spud! A close family friend told me to apply for all my records, which I did. I spent the next six months piecing together what had happened. Night and day, I worked meticulously, comparing hospital records with social services records. I cannot put into words how difficult it was to read all these records, in particular the social worker's records, because of how inaccurate they were. The social worker had an entrenched, negative view in relation to mental health. In her reports she focused on the misdiagnosis of EUPD and made overexaggerated claims about the misdiagnosis, which were not backed up by any medical expert. Her assertion was that an 'oppressive medical professional' within the first mother and baby unit had challenged her about her discriminatory approach (I stumbled across this in the records). I would just like to applaud the bravery of this individual; he was one of the few professionals who made a stand.

Once I had pieced together all the medical evidence, I had to try to get someone to listen to me, which was harder than I thought. In my possession I had clear evidence that I had been set up to fail and that the court had been misled at the time of my daughter's removal. You would have thought that professionals would sit up and listen, but this was definitely not the case. I was told that the circumstances around my daughter's removal were not important and that I should focus on proving that I was a capable parent. I found this hard to digest. Surely the fact that I had evidence to suggest human rights violations had taken place was rather important. I tried to explain to my solicitor at the time how damning this evidence was, but she didn't believe me.

I felt hopeless; the injustice was unbelievable. It wasn't until months later that I had a meeting with my solicitor and the barrister appointed to fight my case. I took my bulging lever-arch folder to that meeting. I sat down with the barrister and showed him all the evidence I had uncovered. His eyes almost popped out of his head as he read through the pages and pages of evidence! He said that this case would be better for his colleague who had more expertise in this area. Finally, someone had listened to what I had to say instead of just seeing the diagnoses, although it would take over a year for my hard work to pay off and my daughter and I to be reunited.

Child in Care meetings

Child in Care (CIC) meetings are supposed to be an opportunity for those involved to have round-the-table discussions about the child in care and the care plan. They are chaired by an independent reviewing officer (IRO), and various professionals who are involved usually attend, for example the social worker, foster carer, child's guardian and so on. Every time I attended a CIC meeting, I felt belittled and intimidated. I often made creative suggestions relating to the care of my daughter which were rubbished by the IRO. These meetings were not an opportunity for discussions about the child; they felt more like an opportunity to disempower me as a parent. I complained many times about the CIC meetings along with other professionals working with me who had never experienced such hostile meetings. Once again, we were ignored. These meetings should have never been allowed to take place.

Child protection

The child protection process was an extremely negative experience for me. When I analyse this, it feels like the stigma associated with being autistic was a barrier alongside the stigma associated with mental health difficulties. Social services were involved for over two years; in all that time not one social worker asked me, 'How does your autism impact your day-to-day life?' Prior to social services involvement, I really believed that they would offer some help and support to ease the transition into motherhood. Unfortunately, this was far from what happened.

I often felt that social services constantly focused on my diagnosis of EUPD, and my autism diagnosis took a back seat. This caused major barriers, and these barriers were often misunderstood as refusal to engage with services or a deterioration in my mental health.

The current child protection system is not working. Children are still dying at the hands of their caregivers, perpetrators slipping through the cracks because they can deceive and manipulate social workers with unrealistic caseloads, whereas, on the flipside, some parents and children are having their rights violated simply because they ask for help. Many of my experiences were echoed within a United Kingdom Human Rights Committee report written by Blakemore (2015), outlining human rights violations against autistic parents: 'No woman should need to consider system failure and rights violations as part of her future reproductive choices' (Blakemore 2015).

I am sad to say that, as an autistic female, I am having to consider my future reproductive choices very carefully. As things stand currently within the UK, I do not feel able to have any more children because of the lack of professional understanding around autistic parents and neurodiverse families and the absence of tailored support.

Forever branded

A number of years have passed since the return of my daughter. When the local authority was ordered to return my daughter, they couldn't close our case quickly enough, which was a stark contrast between the two years they spent apparently setting me up to fail and doing everything in their power to keep us apart.

The child protection process dehumanised me. Even after the full return of my daughter I didn't feel human; I felt worthless. I viewed myself as a slug, despised by many and unwanted: a useless stain on society. I am no longer the same person. I spent two years in fight mode trying to prove my case. Once the decision was made to return my daughter, it was like what on earth had just happened! I had so many questions which remained unanswered.

Life after child protection has been challenging. How does anyone move on from such a traumatic event? Some people have said to me, 'You have got your daughter back, you won', as if my daughter's return removes the damaging trauma we were wrongfully subjected to! Others tell me that time heals all wounds. I hate this saying because the person who came up with this probably never experienced trauma or loss: time doesn't heal all wounds; I am still as hurt as I was when they removed my seven-week-old baby. You can't really move on or heal after suffering such a loss. We cannot turn back time. All those precious memories were denied and cannot be replaced.

For me I had two choices: remain bitter and angry, or forgive the professionals responsible, come to terms with what happened to us and try to make change happen. Forgiveness is an ongoing process. At first it was very difficult, but the more I kept forgiving and letting go, the more tolerable it became. Coming to terms with, and accepting, what has happened to us is also an ongoing journey, and I have to say that turning such a horrific event into something to positively raise awareness has helped us as a family find peace in such painful circumstances.

However, this was not quite the end. I went on to experience further degrading and discriminatory treatment within the family courts. In one example, it was suggested that because I was a single autistic mother at the time, I required a 'normal' partner to balance out my autism-related deficits, so that my child would not be severely damaged by my autism. Somehow this discriminatory language is perfectly acceptable behind closed doors. I feel I have no choice but to continue my education and become a specialist in autism in order to protect myself from these institutions. I am not alone; I am meeting more and more like me – autistic females whose experiences echo mine, all having to become specialists in autism in order to protect themselves and educate others in order to prevent other autistic people from experiencing the same rights violations.

CHAPTER FOUR

Emotionally Unstable Personality Disorder and Autism

This chapter explores both the concept of EUPD in more detail and discusses how it may impact upon those who are given this diagnosis, particularly women. The issue of how this impacts upon both younger and older women will be discussed. Although this chapter refers predominantly to the experiences of females, it is acknowledged that some males and some non-binary individuals also receive this diagnosis, and the impact is no less significant for them.

EUPD is described as a mental illness and appears in the DSM-5 and is used to describe individuals who present with a pattern of unstable personal relationships, often have a very poor self-image, have significant difficulty in regulating their feelings and who tend to behave in an impulsive fashion, and as was briefly discussed in Chapter One, it is one of the key areas where misdiagnosis might occur. There are a number of areas where this type of misdiagnosis can have a significant impact. First, it was not originally intended to be a diagnosis given to anyone under the age of 18, yet it is frequently given in inpatient settings to young women in their teens, under the guise of referring to it as an 'emerging personality disorder'. This is despite the fact that three of the criteria

– 'persistently unstable self-image', 'inappropriate anger' and 'affective instability/rapid mood changes' – could quite possibly be applied to the majority of teenagers and are a normal part of adolescent development!

The second area is the issue of the gendered nature of a EUPD diagnosis. The DSM states certain personality disorders (e.g. antisocial personality disorder) are more frequently diagnosed in males. Others (e.g. borderline, histrionic and dependent personality disorders) are diagnosed more frequently in females. It then goes on to state that although these differences probably reflect genuine gender differences, in the presence of such patterns, clinicians must be cautious not to over or under diagnose certain personality disorders in females or males because of social stereotypes about typical gender roles and behaviour.

In fact, 75 per cent of all diagnoses of EUPD are made in women, and in fact the boys and men I have come across in clinical practice who have received this diagnosis are often undiagnosed autistic, but presenting in a more 'female' way.

Chapman, Jamil and Fleister (2022) report Peter Fonagy *et al.*'s (2017) description of EUPD as 'the result of lack of resilience against psychological stressors'. In the bio-social model, proposed by Dr Marsha Linehan, cited in Crowell, Beauchaine and Linehan (2009), it was agreed that EUPD often emerges as a result of a genetic vulnerability combined with a chronically invalidating environment. However, Kernberg and Michels (2009) tend to focus more upon those who have experienced a pattern of disorganised attachment with a primary caregiver. They cite cases where a parent has behaved in an inconsistent manner, switching (sometimes rapidly) from loving and caring to harsh and punitive, leading the child to struggle with relationships as they grow up.

Regardless of the different theories around how and why personality disorders develop, there is no denying that there is a huge stigma attached to the label.

Ring and Lawn (2019) conducted a study that investigated the stigma associated with having a diagnosis of EUPD from both a patient and professional perspective. They report that psychiatric illnesses in general come with a fair amount of stigma and judgement from society. The impact of admitting to mental health challenges and the resulting prejudice and discrimination that so frequently result can, and do, deter people from seeking support, which can then lead to further exacerbation of difficulties and ultimately to isolation.

A diagnosis of EUPD is perhaps one of the most poorly understood mental health challenges as, superficially, it tends to be perceived as an inability to cope with the challenges of everyday life. It is also the diagnosis that is probably one of the most disputed by medical professionals, who have historically challenged (and continue to challenge) its legitimacy as a 'real' illness. There is a whole narrative about patients being perceived as 'needy', 'manipulative' and 'attention seeking'.

Ring and Lawn (2019) carried out a review of the available literature and concluded that, particularly in inpatient services, those diagnosed with EUPD were made to feel that they were 'wasting people's time' and reported that any complaints or issues they raised were not taken seriously. Others, who were parents, were reluctant to seek help if they needed it with their parenting. Very often, and somewhat worryingly, some patients reported not even being told about their diagnosis face to face and only finding out about it when, and if, they saw their medical notes.

Some professionals acknowledged that they had not had an honest discussion with their patients and tended to refer to EUPD in quite vague, euphemistic, terms, or by referring to other, less stigmatising, diagnoses (such as depression).

Sulzer (2015) also conducted a study exploring how a diagnosis of EUPD was managed by professionals, and outlined the negative consequences of withholding a diagnosis from patients in an attempt to 'protect' them from the stigma, when, in fact, it actually reinforced it in quite a demeaning and paternalistic way.

From this study also came confirmation that individuals with this diagnosis are difficult, or even impossible, to treat. This was partly attributed to a growing demand for support and underlying concerns about the lack of specialist services deemed capable of supporting such a 'complex' group of people. Some health professionals reported in the Sulzer study that they did not feel that providing treatment for EUPD was their responsibility, with certain professional groups (namely registered nurses, mental health nurses and psychiatrists) stating that the overall prognosis for those with a diagnosis was fairly negative. It was also reported that some psychologists also held negative views about the ability of people with EUPD to effect meaningful change in their lives. Sulzer also noted that many mental health professionals reported feeling 'powerless' in the face of extreme distress and find patients who present in this way very difficult to support, leading them to place the emphasis upon 'helping themselves' rather than asking for support when they were struggling.

Bodner *et al.* (2015) carried out a study with psychiatrists exploring negative attitudes towards patients with a diagnosis of EUPD and noted that they too reported feelings of helplessness and impotence when providing treatment. This was found to be strongly correlated with a fear of the patient dying, which is unsurprising given the high rates of suicidality amongst this group. Bodner *et al.* also reported that patients were often referred to as 'selfish' or 'irresponsible', often to their face. Sulzer highlighted how this type of attitude can very easily lead to the emphasis shifting from the patient having a mental illness, to simply displaying 'bad behaviour', thus moving the focus away from EUPD personality being a medical issue.

This then raises the issue of autistic people who receive this diagnosis. The first issue is whether it is appropriate to jump to the conclusion that the individual has a 'personality disorder' rather than fully exploring their autism and the impact of a lifetime of being misunderstood. Second, when this does happen, what are the implications for individuals labelled in this way, both for younger people, who receive a diagnosis as a teenager, and for those who are missed (or misdiagnosed) and who present with mental health challenges throughout their adult life?

May *et al.* (2021) go on to outline that, overall, several features which are present in those with a EUPD diagnosis are also seen in those with a diagnosis of autism. They cite, for example, difficulties in interpreting the thoughts, feelings and actions of others; difficulties reading facial expression; and sensory issues (which were added to the autism criteria when the DSM-5 was published in 2013; APA 2013). They also cite the high levels of self-harm and suicidal behaviour that have been reported, particularly in autistic girls and women (Hedley and Uljarevic 2018), and issues around identity. In fact, the only area where there was not a strong similarity between EUPD and autism was in the restrictive and repetitive interests domain, and many autistic females do not score highly in this area anyway.

However, returning to the original point, viewing behaviours as symptoms or features of a disorder – without taking into account triggers or other features that may have contributed to the development of what is, essentially, a trauma or distress response – seems short-sighted. Especially when bearing in mind the stigma that a diagnosis of personality disorder attracts. It is easy to see why so many autistic women are diagnosed when the externalising behaviour is, on the surface, very similar. Where the problems really begin, though, is when mental health professionals dismiss an existing diagnosis of autism (or strong suggestions in a person's history that might point to autism being an appropriate diagnosis). This can not only lead to the individual feeling invalidated, it can also, wrongly, place the 'blame' for the development of these difficulties upon the close family. What this means in reality is that not only are young (and older) people placed in inpatient units far from home, they are also often isolated from their families. In addition, the environment and the treatment programme are unlikely to meet their needs.

AYLA'S STORY

Ayla was loyal, honest, generous, selfless and compassionate. She loved her home and family and had a close relationship with her mother and grandmother. She had a natural affinity with animals. She loved outdoor activities and sport and was passionate about karate. She was adventurous and had a great sense of fun. She always considered others before herself and brought out the best in people. Ayla learnt to cook at an early age. She would spend many hours drawing and colouring and had a talent for creative writing.

Ayla started secondary school when she was 11 and found the transition difficult and highly stressful. She began to self-harm at home by using a razor to shave layers of skin off her leg. Ayla could not understand the dynamics of a bigger school, and the social context appeared to be too much for her to cope with.

In 2006 a detailed report was commissioned by Ayla's school from an educational psychologist who noted that Ayla displayed traits of autism.

Hospital admissions

At the age of 15 years Ayla developed obsessional thoughts around food intake. Ayla also withdrew from her peers, disengaged socially and found it too difficult to engage in the usual activities that teenagers would normally enjoy. It became apparent that she was struggling with her eating, and there were times when she wanted to eat but would throw away her food. Ayla became restrictive in terms of what she would and would not eat. She would also exercise a great deal.

She was eventually admitted to hospital for nasogastric feeding and was diagnosed with anorexia nervosa. Ayla stayed in hospital intermittently for approximately the next 18 months. Here she was prescribed antipsychotics for the first time, including Olanzapine and Fluoxetine. Olanzapine appeared to result in considerable side effects. Ayla presented as depressed and began to dribble excessively. She also started walking with an unstable gait and seemed generally disconnected from her surroundings. Her responsible clinician at the time told Ayla's mother that he did not know what was wrong with her other than anorexia nervosa, so the family decided to consult with a local psychologist privately to assess Ayla. The report concluded that Ayla had dysexecutive problems and clinicians should be careful not to confuse this with EUPD. This report was unfortunately never acknowledged and was later discredited.

Adult mental health services

After two incidents of self-harm at home (that professionals considered to be suicide attempts), Ayla went into an acute adult inpatient unit. While the team was focusing on the episodes of self-harm that had led to her admission, her anorexia diagnosis was often overlooked.

Ayla's mother did not feel that the treatment plan implemented by the hospital was working. It was based on a reward-style programme where Ayla would have things taken away from her if she did not do 'well'.

As a result of her inability to settle, and an increase in what was described as 'challenging behaviour', Ayla was subsequently moved to a low secure forensic unit (70 miles away from her home). It was at this point that Ayla's aggression increased significantly, and she was put in seclusion in a converted bathroom with a mattress on a concrete floor where she stayed for ten months. Ayla's responsible clinician later requested that Ayla be transferred to another unit. One of the reasons given was the family's interference. They had also been told on a previous occasion to 'leave it to the medical professionals – we are her family now'!

Whilst Ayla was detained, two consultant forensic psychiatrists were asked to assess Ayla for the purpose of finding a suitable placement and management and whether detention in a medium secure unit was warranted. The responsible clinician commented: 'The current scenario of Ayla and the family unit being enmeshed could be ameliorated, in part, by some physical distance.' He also stated that the 'current approach is not working'. Another recommendation was that she should be dealt with by the judicial system. Despite his recommendation that a move to a medium secure unit would only perpetuate Ayla's behaviours, she was transferred to a medium secure unit (220 miles from home). Several attempts were made to prevent Ayla being placed in a medium secure environment and so far away from home. These attempts included central government involvement, but at the time there was considered to be no other option.

At this time, one of the doctors from Ayla's home team looked at the notes and requested a consultant psychiatrist in learning disabilities and autism spectrum disorder (ASD) interview with Ayla's mother and grandmother about her past behaviours to clarify if a specialist assessment for ASD was indicated as he had observed the many references to autism in Ayla's developmental history. The result of the assessment was that Ayla had obvious traits of autism that should be further explored. However, another doctor at the hospital categorically denied that Ayla was autistic because she was 'too warm and friendly'. She also stated that she felt the health board had acted unprofessionally in requesting the report. At this time, Ayla was also prescribed excessive medication with obvious side effects and no known benefit. She had no choice in this. There is sufficient documented evidence to show that many of the drugs prescribed had failed. A trial of Clozapine was commenced but had to be stopped abruptly because of the side effects resulting in Ayla having to be placed in seclusion for 10 days. Her prescribed medication appeared to be far removed from the NICE guidelines.

Due to continued deterioration the family were informed that a suggestion had been made to refer Ayla to a high secure hospital (Rampton), but this was refused. The family were informed that Ayla's responsible clinician had requested a referral assessment from Rampton Hospital, but it was refused. Ayla's presentation began to deteriorate again. Her view of hospital life was sadly that she had little prospect of hope and that she could not see a way forward that would see her resuming even a small part of the life she once had. At times, she was made to sit on a beanbag facing the wall for a whole day as a punishment. The family complained to the social worker who informed them that he would report the incident to the safeguarding team. No referral was made. The family believe that many efforts were made to discredit and alienate Ayla from them including cancelling visits for over 12 months.

Her own journal during August 2021 shows the heart-breaking struggle she had with her physical and mental health and her homesickness.

She regularly suffered psychotic episodes and would see snakes in the corner of the room. She would frequently disassociate and have non-epileptic fits.

Ayla took her own life earlier this year whilst still in hospital. She never made it back home again.

Assessment for autism

Ayla's mother had always believed that she was autistic, but throughout her life professionals refused to carry out an assessment. She offered to pay to have an independent assessment but was informed that the doctors would never accept the result. Ayla never had an assessment for autism.

Ayla's story is truly tragic, and she is not the only young person to be failed in this way by a system that does not understand them. Her family are bravely sharing her story in the hope that, by doing so, change will happen.

I also received similar stories from adult women who were diagnosed with EUPD and who were actually simply autistic women in a world that made no allowances for them.

JENNY'S STORY

Jenny did not receive her diagnosis of autism and ADHD until she was in her late 50s and describes a lifetime of feeling 'misunderstood' and getting things 'wrong'. She talks articulately about how she would dress in her late teens and how, as an attractive young woman who had not fitted in or felt popular during her teenage years, she began wearing clothing that, in her own words, could have been described as 'slutty' or 'seductive', but without really understanding either, and recalls many occasions where she totally misread the intentions of the men who paid her attention. This pattern of vulnerability has been described elsewhere in this book and in my previous book (Eaton 2017) and is a pattern that is repeated frequently, often with appalling outcomes. Jenny also referred to her ongoing social communication difficulties and feelings of shame. In an attempt to overcome these, she reported beginning to use alcohol as a social facilitator and admitted to often ending up in unwanted sexual situations in her search for comfort and acceptance. She ultimately went to see a psychiatrist who diagnosed her with clinical depression and prescribed medication. Shortly after, she describes her first suicide attempt where she took an overdose of paracetamol and aspirin. After having her stomach pumped and being told that she had, in fact, taken enough medication to kill herself, she then accepted a voluntary admission to a psychiatric ward. During this admission, Jenny acknowledges adopting various 'personas', wearing different clothes and trying a variety of identities, presumably as a way of trying to both find out who she really was and as a further attempt to fit in.

During this admission, after bravely opening up about her sexual vulnerability, her psychiatrist diagnosed her with hypersexuality. She also reported that sometime later, when she visited a family planning clinic, she told the nurse of this diagnosis without having any idea of the stigma involved with such an admission. This provides a further insight into the subtle, but devastating, impact of autistic communication challenges as she simply did not realise how this admission would be received by others. When she eventually realised, she describes feeling 'shamefully embarrassed', which is a theme that occurs time and time again in her story.

Once released from hospital, Jenny stopped taking her medication, and, following the example of a new friend, she began restricting her food intake and using diuretics and laxatives in an attempt to manage her weight. She describes this as 'wanting to disappear and be in control' and also reports wanting to be 'impervious to criticism' as she felt that this would happen if she became slimmer. Her whole life at this point was about desperately trying to achieve perfection. This resulted ultimately in a second psychiatric admission. During this admission she reported having been referred to as a 'nuisance' and an 'attention seeker'. Shortly after, she was given a diagnosis of EUPD, which she accepted as she had no idea what it meant. In some ways, she reported feeling relieved because, at last, there was a name for what was 'wrong' with her.

Following this and her subsequent release from hospital, Jenny continued to experience a number of challenges. Like many autistic women, when she became pregnant she did not have an enjoyable pregnancy and also reported that her son was wrongly removed from her care (he was later diagnosed as autistic). She goes on to describe her eventual diagnosis of autism and ADHD as a process of 'adjustment and acceptance'.

Throughout her story, the overriding theme is one of misunderstanding, combined with high levels of guilt and shame. She also reports a lifetime of masking and trying to fit in.

People often question why someone would seek a diagnosis late in life, and Jenny's story is a wonderful example of how a diagnosis can lead to peace and acceptance and having the confidence to be her authentic self.

So, was her initial diagnosis of EUPD justified? Possibly, at the time, given that this diagnosis is essentially a description of someone in distress. However, would an earlier diagnosis have changed how she felt about herself, or how others judged her? As a vulnerable young woman, growing up in a world of judgement and where anyone who is 'different' can be bullied and made to feel bad about themselves, possibly not. Young autistic people growing up today in a world where social media dominates their lives, and it seems to be even more unacceptable to be different, may find life even harder. However, what today's society does offer is a greater opportunity for people to connect with other neurodiverse people and to essentially find their 'tribe'. Jenny now enjoys life, is her authentic self, and is accepted and liked by her family and friends for who she is.

This does not take away the need for better understanding of the needs of autistic people as they age. There are likely to be many undiagnosed autistic adults whose needs have not been explored. An article by Mason *et al.* (2022) reported the findings of a review of the literature into the experiences of older autistic adults. They found that older adult studies accounted for only 0.4 per cent of all published studies about autism from the last decade. They did, however, note that there has been a positive upward trend over the last few years. They concluded that more research was needed into the practical aspects of autistic life, such as social isolation, living arrangements and the needs of older adults with intellectual disability.

A study, published in 2017 (Autistica 2017), highlighted that autistic people die, on average, 16 years before their non-autistic peers, with autistic people without a learning disability being nine times more likely to die from suicide.

In addition to mental health challenges, autistic people are statistically more likely to experience poor health including cardiovascular disease, diabetes, stroke, and circulatory and respiratory conditions. The reasons for this are not entirely clear, but the Autistica study did note the following:

- Autistic people can have a more restricted diet, may take less exercise and may be prescribed more medication than non-autistic people.
- They may face social pressures, such as bullying, pressure to conform to societal ideals and experience social isolation.

- They are likely to experience high levels of anxiety, depression and sensory overload.

And perhaps, crucially:

- Autistic people can face significant barriers to accessing health care.

This is before considering other factors that may impact upon autistic adults as they age, such as the menopause and failing cognitive ability or dementia.

There is clearly a need for better understanding both by society and primary and secondary health care providers of the challenges faced by autistic persons as they age, and this once again highlights the risks of missed or misdiagnosis.

CHAPTER FIVE

Missed or Misdiagnosis in the Classroom

This chapter will explore the implications of a missed or misdiagnosis in the classroom, with particular consideration of instances where the reported behaviour(s) are not seen at school and where the relationship between school and parents breaks down.

The issue of masking or 'social camouflaging' in autistic people has been mentioned in previous chapters, specifically in relation to diagnosis and ongoing mental health challenges. Chapter One also explored the diagnostic process for children and young people and discussed the suggestions in the NICE guidelines for the assessment and diagnosis of autism spectrum disorders in under 19s (NICE 2017), that information regarding a child or young person's functioning is gathered from a third-party source. Often this third-party source, particularly in the case of younger children, is the child's school or educational placement. So, what happens if a child is presenting at home with significant distress and/or challenging behaviour, but as far as school staff are concerned, there are no problems? What if the child is described in school as a 'model student' who is apparently coping well in the classroom, is sociable and communicates well with both teachers and peers?

Basically, if the assessment team in the area where the child or young person lives insists upon corroboration of difficulties from the school setting, this can (and often does) result in the assessment request, or referral, not being accepted. In some cases, this can even lead to accusations of poor parenting. Comments are often made about the child's attachment and parental boundaries (or perceived lack of them). In a worst-case scenario, this may lead to the parent being subjected to child protection proceedings (especially if the child begins to refuse to attend school) or even accusations of FII. (This is discussed in further detail in Chapters Eight and Nine.) One mother's story (itmustbemum 2017) highlights the issues that can occur when staff within a child's school fail to accept a diagnosis of autism from professional(s) appropriately trained and experienced in the area.

One child's story

For this child, he went from being an autistic child, who, with the right level of support and understanding, could quite possibly have achieved well in a mainstream primary school setting, to a child who needed Tier 4 (inpatient) assessment, and who thus became a child with 'complex' needs.

The story begins at the point that the child was assessed and given a diagnosis of Asperger's Syndrome (the diagnostic category used at the time). His mother then arranged to speak with the headteacher, to establish what support could be put in place for him. She reports that she was met with the assertion that he was 'normal' and that maybe there was an issue with his attachment. The school special educational needs coordinator (SENCO) subsequently carried out her own 'observation' of the child, and she too determined that the child was 'fine'. There followed a three-year refusal to offer support, details of which only became apparent during a subject access request (SAR).

However, the child's mental health declined rapidly, and he went from being a child in a mainstream school without support to being in an inpatient service and assessed as needing a specialist residential placement.

The child's mother then contacted their local authority special educational needs manager to pass on the information gathered at the child's Care Programme Approach (CPA) meeting at the hospital. She assumed that this would trigger a change in his Education, Health and

Care Plan (EHCP), the draft of which was due soon. She was then told that it was just 'one person's opinion' (despite the fact that it was the view of a multi-agency team following a six-week assessment period in an inpatient unit).

The hospital report confirmed his diagnosis, which in addition to Asperger's Syndrome now included additional mental health diagnoses such as mixed anxiety-depressive disorder and highlighted 'serious social disability'.

The child's mother further reports that from the time of his initial referral to CAMHS four-and-a-half years previously he had been under the care of five psychiatrists and two paediatricians, not to mention a variety of other clinicians, all highly experienced in neurodevelopmental difficulties. He had a well-established and long-standing diagnosis of autism, provided by appropriately qualified and experienced professionals.

However, the child's mother then goes on to report that staff within the child's school continued to believe that the medical teams were wrong. She expresses her concern about how teaching staff, with no significant training in either mental health or neurodevelopmental disorders, could simply overrule a diagnosis and consequent recommendations.

At the point of her son's discharge from the inpatient unit, the child's mother then had only six weeks to organise his school placement. He still had no EHCP, and no local authority educational psychologist had been allocated to assess him.

Masking in the school environment

Mandy (2019) describes the process of 'masking' or social camouflaging in adults. Adults are clearly better able to articulate their motivation for masking or attempting to hide the fact that they are autistic. However, it is safe to assume that many children will also adopt the same approach and for the same reasons.

Mandy reports on the high number of autistic individuals who invest huge effort, daily, attempting to modify and adapt their behaviour to fit in with non-autistic norms and expectations. This can involve, for example, suppressing or hiding 'stims' or repetitive movements that the individual enjoys or finds comforting, using eye contact in a socially appropriate manner, or actively studying and imitating the behaviour of their non-autistic peers, in the hope of fitting in and not standing out or appearing 'different'.

One study (cited by Mandy 2019) by Cage and Troxell-Whitman (2019) reported that 70 per cent of the autistic participants in their study reported having consciously camouflaged or hidden their true identity. A study by Hull *et al.* (2017) noted that autistic persons masked in order to avoid bullying, whilst others felt that it helped them to negotiate the education system and the workplace and make friends.

This masking does, however, come with an increased risk of distress. Constantly being on high alert and internalising distress and discomfort can lead to either higher levels of anxiety or the 'meltdowns' that are so commonly reported when children and young people return to the safety and security of their homes.

Mandy further reports that the study of camouflaging or masking in autistic adults highlights the role of the environment in the development of many of the challenges experienced by both autistic children and adults, and states that for too long it has been assumed that difficulties arise because of deficits in the autistic person, rather than appreciating the demands that the environment puts on them.

The autistic cognitive profile

In a school environment, the need to mask and fit in with peers is only one aspect of how an autistic child may try to stay 'beneath the radar' at school.

It is well known that many autistic children (without a clear intellectual difficulty) have what is referred to as a 'spiky' cognitive profile, indicating that there are likely to be distinct areas of strength and difficulty. A recent study by Audras-Torrent *et al.* (2021) confirmed my own clinical experience. This study found that, overall, the cohort of children they assessed with the WISC V (The Wechsler Intelligence Scale for Children, version V) achieved significantly lower scores in sub-tests that measured their working memory and processing speed compared to their verbal comprehension scores. Further they found that the children's auditory working memory was poorer than their visual working memory.

So, how does this impact upon the way in which a child may present in the classroom? First, it is likely that the child will be relatively articulate and verbally able (the caveat to this being those young people who are selectively mute at school). However, if their working memory and processing speed are significantly poorer, this can have a major impact upon their school performance and is often attributed to 'laziness' or 'lack of attention'. In reality it can make attending to instructions almost impossible. When this is combined with visual processing difficulties or poor visual motor integration (which can make it very difficult for the child to get their thoughts down on paper quickly), it is clear to see how problems might arise in the classroom, which might not be obvious to the casual observer, particularly if the child is trying not to stand out or get into trouble. Many autistic children also experience significant challenges with their executive functioning – these are the operations needed for good planning, organisation, task shifting and sequencing. This may explain why so many autistic children are not identified until they start high school and are able to manage reasonably well at primary school. The transition to high school involves changing from one teacher teaching the class, generally in one room for the whole day, to multiple teachers teaching across a school site. Imagine the scenario – a teacher (verbally) gives instructions to the class about homework and may also write something on the board for the children to copy. Both of these tasks would be a challenge for an autistic child with difficulties in this area. They then have to move quickly to their next lesson – making sure they have the right books and equipment and can find their way easily to the next class. Many parents report that their children 'hold it together' whilst at school and do not display their confusion or distress, only to break down at home, or even begin to avoid or refuse school.

This is all in addition to potential friendship issues, bullying, sensory overload and the fact that the school curriculum becomes increasingly complex and abstract at high school. So, when a teacher claims that a child is 'fine' in school and all they see is an apparently able child who, in their eyes, displays no signs of autism, it is important to reflect that behaviour is a form of communication. Difficult, or challenging, behaviour in the home may not reflect poor parental boundaries or 'attachment' problems, and in fact putting in place fairly simple interventions once the child's strengths and difficulties are identified may help to avoid this type of issue.

CHAPTER SIX

Autism in the Family Courts, Inpatient Services and Criminal Justice System

This chapter will provide an introduction to the issues that can arise following a misdiagnosis or failure to diagnose an autism spectrum condition and will include examples from mental health services and family court proceedings.

Parenting assessments and the family courts

'Parenting Assessment Frameworks' were developed to help social workers who have concerns about a parent's ability to meet the needs of their child.

The London Borough of Southwark Safeguarding Service Parenting Assessment Framework (London Borough of Southwark 2016) promotes the use of a 'systematic, evidence based and analytical' approach which can be used to identify perceived risks, strengths and protective factors and which allows social work practitioners to reach a clear and structured judgement about whether an individual has the 'capacity' to meet the needs of their child.

The term 'parenting capacity' was used in the Department of Health Framework for the Assessment of Children in Need and Their Families (2000) and included the following:

- Basic care: providing for a child's physical and dental needs.
- Ensuring safety: ensuring the child is adequately protected from harm or danger.
- Emotional warmth: ensuring the child's emotional needs are met and the child feels valued.
- Stimulation: promoting the child's learning and intellectual development, through encouragement, cognitive stimulation and promoting social opportunities.
- Guidance and boundaries: enabling the child to regulate their own emotions and behaviour – with the key parental tasks being demonstrating and modelling appropriate behaviour and control of emotions and interactions with others, and setting boundaries so the child is able to develop an internal model of moral values, conscience and appropriate social behaviour.
- Stability: providing a sufficiently stable family environment to enable the child to develop secure attachments to their caregiver.

Endeavouring to ensure all the above needs are met can be difficult when a child is autistic: a child who, for example, lacks a basic sense of danger and who may be prone to impulsive actions or running away from their caregiver, who struggles to regulate their emotions, who may be prone to sudden and explosive 'meltdowns', and who does not share the same need for social interaction with others. Some children may also struggle to take care (or be supported to take care) of their basic hygiene and dental needs. Many autistic children have sensory needs that impact upon their ability to tolerate tooth brushing or even the food they are prepared to eat.

All the above could be interpreted as 'significant issues' by a social work practitioner. This is particularly true when, for whatever reason, a child is not accurately assessed or diagnosed, or when there is significant disagreement about a diagnostic label.

Many parents, when struggling to manage sometimes challenging behaviour, will initially reach out to their local social care team for support and advice. It is easy to see how many of the aspects covered in the criteria for determining 'good enough' parenting could be mis-interpreted as the parents not coping, or not being willing to impose appropriate boundaries.

However, the reason why a parent might be struggling should not automatically be seen as them lacking capacity or not having a clear understanding of the need for basic parenting guidelines. Most of the parents who struggle with this type of challenge are caring, loving and well informed, and whilst in a transactional relationship it is never appropriate to 'blame' the child, many years of clinical experience has shown me that some children are temperamentally more complex to support. Simply parent blaming does not help either the parents or the young person.

Insisting that a young person should attend school every day, for example, when the environment might be traumatic for them, both from a sensory and an academic perspective, is surely unethical and is unlikely to result in a good outcome.

Issues can, and do, arise when social work practitioners are not sufficiently well informed about the complex nature of some autistic children and young people's support needs.

The following case represents an amalgam of a number of cases that have gone to court and highlights how a request for support for a difficult home situation can quickly escalate into accusations of poor or inadequate parenting.

Child A

Child A was the fourth child out of six children born to Mr and Mrs B. They lived in an intact family. There was a family history of neurodi-versity. However, all of Mr and Mrs B's other children were reported to be doing well. All were attending school, and none were subject to a child in need or a child protection plan.

From an early age, Child A began to display behaviour that was described as challenging. This often took the form of violent and uncontrollable 'meltdowns' that were usually triggered when someone said 'no' to her or she was prevented from having, or doing, what she wanted. Her language development had been good, and there were no obvious learning difficulties. In addition to daily 'meltdowns' Child A was not sleeping well. She found it almost impossible to settle, and most nights were disturbed for the family.

Mr and Mrs B were experienced parents, well used to implementing guidelines and boundaries, which their other children were able to follow. However, they quickly found that taking the same approach with Child A simply led to more 'meltdowns'. The strategies they had used with their other children did not work and, in fact, made things worse. Ultimately, this resulted in Child A hitting out at, and injuring, both of her parents. In addition, she had also begun to target one of her siblings. She began to tell lies and frequently accused her parents of hurting her (when they were not). Ultimately, they asked their local social care team for support.

Instead of receiving the hoped-for practical and non-judgemental support, Mr and Mrs B found themselves being accused of physical and emotional abuse and Child A was made the subject of an interim care order and placed in emergency foster care.

When the foster carers also reported similar challenges when trying to support Child A, it was finally suggested that she might be autistic and that many of the challenges she, and her family, had experienced could be explained by undiagnosed autism. She was subsequently assessed and diagnosed. However, the family were left feeling broken and unsupported and, to date, Child A remains accommodated away from her parents. Mr and Mrs B now have a permanent question mark over their parenting.

This scenario is not unusual, and unfortunately it is common for parents to be faced in court by solicitors, judges and social workers who simply do not understand autism.

The situation is further complicated in cases which go to the family court when parents have separated and who may have different viewpoints about the difficulties faced by their child. Too often it can result in 'point scoring' where parents wish to blame each other for the challenges. In child arrangement cases, this can lead to disputes which are difficult to resolve.

Louise Desrosiers, a barrister who works in the family court, reported that anecdotal reports pointed to a very high rate of relationship breakdown when parents have an autistic child (Desrosiers 2015).

Desrosiers provides advice for parents who find themselves in this situation. First, she says, it is important to highlight to their legal representative and judge at the beginning of proceedings that there is a suspicion that the child might be autistic. It can then be possible to delay proceedings until an assessment has taken place. Psychological/medical and educational reports can then all be considered.

When there is a dispute between the parties, a report from CAF-CASS (Children and Family Court Advisory and Support Service) can be requested. This report should be independent, and it is important that the expert chosen to complete the report has sufficient knowledge of autism to be able to provide an informed opinion. In cases where there are significant disputes between parents, it can be advisable to ask for a guardian to be appointed to look after the interests of the child. This could be especially pertinent where the difficulties observed by one parent (usually the one who spends most time with the child) are not seen (or acknowledged) by the non-resident parent.

It does, however, remain extremely challenging when parents simply cannot agree. As a clinician, I have been faced with this situation numerous times. For a diagnosis of autism to be given, a comprehensive developmental history needs to be taken. When parents are in dispute this can be a time-consuming and frustrating task and one which makes it impossible to confirm a diagnosis, even though it is quite obvious that this would be appropriate. Ultimately, I would urge any parents who find themselves in this situation, or any professionals working with a family who have polar opposite views, to consider very carefully what is in the best interests of that particular child or young person. Mis- or missed diagnosis remains a significant cause of children being perceived as 'complex'.

'Complex' presentations and the Mental Health Act

In cases where the young person's presentation becomes severely dys-regulated it can also, in some cases, lead to them being detained under the Mental Health Act. A number of high-profile cases have come to light in recent years of young people with 'complex' presentations being detained in mental health facilities, often for long periods of time. These young people are often autistic.

A typical progression into increasingly high levels of security and concern would be for the young person initially to display some form of 'challenging' behaviour at home or at school. This might include anything from violence and aggression towards parents/siblings (as in the case of Child A) where parents have sought support from services, through to incidents of threat, stalking or otherwise risky (to self or others) behaviour which has taken place in the wider community.

Parents, and others involved with the child or young person, may feel they have no choice but to call for police assistance. This can result in the young person being detained under section 136 of the Mental Health Act, which is a brief 'holding' section whereby a young person can be taken to a safe environment to protect themselves and others. Some psychiatric hospitals have dedicated 136 suites, but if one of these is not readily available, the young person may be detained in a cell at a local police station. Once temporarily detained, the young person can be held for up to 72 hours whilst a mental health assessment is arranged. This is usually carried out by two suitably experienced and qualified doctors and an approved mental health practitioner (AMHP), often a social worker. The decision can then be made to admit the young person into hospital for an assessment period of 28 days (known as a Section 2 detention). This usually takes place in a psychiatric intensive care unit (PICU). During this assessment period, if the person is autistic (diagnosed or not), it is not unusual for their behaviour and presentation to become more dysregulated. The change in routine, combined with uncertainty about the future and possible sensory-processing difficulties, can lead to an increase in what are referred to as 'challenging behaviours'. At this point, if their needs are not appropriately assessed, it is quite possible then for the Mental Health section to be extended, and there have been cases where the treating clinicians have felt it necessary to recommend that the young person be moved to a more secure environment.

Sadly, from this point, it is not unusual for the young person to be 'managed' rather than supported (and treated), and some young people find themselves placed in seclusion suites and, in some cases, are denied contact with their peers or members of staff because of their perceived risk to themselves or others.

This, combined with the possibility of being restrained or held (to prevent harm to self or others), can lead to the young person experiencing trauma and flashbacks for years to come.

In addition, at the point of being admitted to a psychiatric unit, even if this has not been part of the young person's treatment up until that point, it is very likely that they will be given medication. Many medications are routinely used to 'manage' the behavioural and emotional challenges of autistic children and young people, including stimulants (such as Methylphenidate) and specific serotonin reuptake inhibitors (SSRIs) which are given to manage anxiety and depression. Some young people are also prescribed antipsychotic medication, particularly if they are presenting with highly aggressive behaviour. It is important to note that not all the young people will necessarily have been displaying aggressive behaviour prior to their hospital admission. However, there is relatively little evidence in the medical literature which examines the potentially different way in which an autistic child or young person might react to this type of medication.

The case study below clearly illustrates this point.

OLIVER'S STORY

Oliver was a young teenager who sadly experienced two episodes of meningitis as a newborn baby which left him with mild hemiplegia, focal partial epilepsy, a mild learning disability and a diagnosis of autism.

Despite these challenges, Oliver grew up into a determined young man who achieved GCSEs and was a talented footballer and track athlete.

He began to experience an increase in his partial focal seizures and, quite understandably, became anxious. He was prescribed antidepressant medication and was subsequently given antipsychotics, despite not having a mental health illness or psychosis. This was reported to have had a catastrophic impact upon Oliver's mood and presentation, and ultimately he was sectioned under the Mental Health Act for assessment. When in hospital it was determined that he was intolerant to antipsychotic medication, and this was stopped.

Sometime later, he was again admitted to hospital with seizures and, once again, prescribed antipsychotic medication. Oliver's parents strongly believe that this, as before, contributed to a decline in his mood and presentation. However, the treating team had very little, or no, understanding of autism when impacted by seizure activity.

He was transferred to an adult general hospital at the request of his parents, which they believed would have a better understanding of his epilepsy. Sadly, this hospital had very little understanding of autism. They did not realise the impact of his sensory difficulties or how overwhelmed he was. He was subsequently restrained on multiple occasions when in seizure by significant numbers of support staff (due to the fact that Oliver needed to walk around, which was a normal part of his seizure presentation). He was also denied any privacy and was not allowed to sleep alone or use the bathroom in private.

Oliver was once again detained under the Mental Health Act and was transferred to a specialist PICU, which thankfully had a better understanding of autism. Their assessment concluded that Oliver was not mentally unwell, and there was no evidence of psychosis. They reduced his antipsychotic medication and discharged him with a letter stressing his intolerance to both antipsychotics and benzodiazepines. He continued to make good progress and was well supported by a specialist community team who understood his autism.

Tragically though, he was once again admitted to hospital following an increase in his seizures and, again, given antipsychotics, despite his family and Oliver himself explaining that he had previously had an adverse reaction to these drugs. Oliver developed neuroleptic malignant syndrome (which caused his brain to swell and resulted in irreparable brain damage), and he died a few days later. An independent learning disability mortality review concluded that Oliver's death was avoidable. It went on to make 35 recommendations to the NHS, which were all accepted.

Oliver's mother, Paula, has campaigned tirelessly since Oliver's untimely death. She feels that the professionals treating him never made any attempt to understand his autism or adapt the environment to meet his needs, relying instead upon medication and restraint. Further information about Oliver's story and the campaign led by his mother Paula can be found online.[1]

1   www.olivermcgowan.org

CHAPTER SEVEN

The Criminal Justice System – Autism, Probation, Risk Assessments and Treatment

This chapter will explore the issue and experiences of autistic individuals who come into contact with the CJS, with specific reference to how treatment plans/probation and risk assessments may change as a result of either getting an autism diagnosis, or alternatively correcting a misdiagnosis.

It will first explore the issue of the potential vulnerability to exploitation of autistic individuals and look at some of the risk factors involved in terms of the possibility of becoming involved in the CJS. The second part of the chapter focuses more upon occasions where autistic individuals actually commit a crime and how being autistic can be considered when formulating probation and risk assessments and when putting together treatment plans.

Autism, vulnerability and the CJS

When a dreadful crime (a mass shooting, or a terrorist attack) takes place, it is often mentioned, almost as an aside, that the perpetrator was autistic or had been identified as a 'loner' with 'autistic traits'. This might lead the general public to assume that being autistic puts a person at additional risk of being involved in a crime. However, the evidence does not support this assertion. Brewer and Young (2018) attribute this in part to the myths and (often incorrect) stereotypes that surround autism. In addition, the assumption is often made that anyone who is a little 'quirky' or different is somewhere on the autistic 'spectrum'. Brewer and Young provide the example of Adam Lanza who went into an American elementary school with a gun and shot 26 people, including 20 children between the ages of six and seven and six members of staff, before killing himself. He had previously shot and killed his mother before driving to the school. He was posthumously diagnosed (by the media) as being autistic, despite not having been formally diagnosed by any professional. This appears to have been based solely upon reports that he was a 'loner' and 'socially awkward'. This raises important issues with regard to autistic people who become involved in the CJS.

Unfortunately, good-quality studies formally examining the incidence of autistic young people being involved in crime are sparse. Many of the studies that are available involved only a small number of participants, had issues regarding how the samples were selected or failed to take into account other factors such as socio-economic status or pre-existing mental health difficulties.

What may be more pertinent, rather than focusing upon the number of individuals with a diagnosis of autism who come into contact with the CJS, would be to explore factors which might make an autistic person more vulnerable to being drawn into criminal activities or to become the victim of exploitation.

One factor which Brewer and Young did discuss was bullying, citing a statistic of over 50 per cent of autistic adult offenders who had been subject to bullying. This was felt to contribute to mood disorders and violence in some cases.

Brewer and Young also suggest that, potentially, 'theory of mind' deficits may lead to a reduced ability to appreciate the impact of one's actions on others and to understand how actions may make another person feel.

The whole issue of 'theory of mind' is highly contentious within the autistic community with critical autism researchers such as Damian Milton (Milton 2012) re-framing theory of mind deficits as a 'double empathy' problem, stating: 'Autism has been positioned as a neurological disorder, a pathological deviance from expected functional stages of development' (p.883). Basically, Milton is arguing for a different way of thinking about neurodiversity, namely that it is not simply a case of the autistic person not understanding the neurotypical (non-autistic) way of thinking and social norms, but more accurately a mismatch in understanding from both sides – the neurotypical often fails to appreciate how the autistic person thinks, feels and rationalises decisions.

My own clinical experience in this regard is somewhat mixed. There is no doubt that the myth of all autistic people being unable to empathise or see a situation from another person's point of view is clearly untrue. I have observed, worked with and supported many autistic individuals who are highly empathetic.

However, when working in forensic inpatient services and more recently, when involved in carrying out autism diagnostic assessments in prison settings, I have seen clear evidence of some autistic individuals finding it extremely challenging (or even impossible) to shift from a particular viewpoint about something (or someone) and failing to appreciate the wider impact of their actions. This can make rehabilitation work difficult and can make those working with such individuals (and those making decisions about whether they are ready for release from a mental health section, or parole) come to the conclusion that the person lacks empathy and is uncaring about the impact of their actions on their victim(s). It is possible, therefore, that challenges may increase exponentially alongside the degree of inflexibility in the individual's thinking, which is itself on a spectrum and does not exclusively impact upon autistic people.

Another factor which may contribute to a potential vulnerability to becoming involved in criminal activity, or to financial, emotional or sexual exploitation, is the presence of comorbid conditions such as ADHD, which may lead to more impulsive behaviour and additional difficulties in thinking ahead and considering possible consequences for actions.

In real-life terms, it may be helpful to imagine the scenario of a group of young people engaging in a petty crime, such as minor acts of vandalism. It is nearly always the vulnerable individual who is left 'holding the brick' when the police arrive, as the other young people are more likely to have read the situation better and run off. This then raises the question of how these vulnerable young people are managed when they do come into contact with the police and the wider criminal justice system.

Autism, radicalisation and terrorism

There is limited empirical evidence to suggest that autistic persons may be vulnerable to becoming engaged in terrorist activities. However, a paper by Al-Attar (2020) outlines some of the potential risks for autistic people and adds further evidence to the argument that, if individuals remain undiagnosed, or misdiagnosed, these risks may not be evaluated. Al-Attar is keen to point out that it is important to avoid stigmatising autistic persons and that the risks may be contextual rather than causal – put simply, it might be that certain autistic features *may* shape a person's experience, how they function and socialise and how this may lead to increased vulnerability. The paper further explored the social and eco-logical factors that may also serve to 'push' an individual towards terror-ist groups and ideology, and the first factor identified was circumscribed interests. Autistic people often spend many hours researching topics of interest in great detail. Anthony *et al.* (2013) also highlighted how the intensity of 'special interests' may lead autistic persons to hyperfocus, sometimes to an extreme degree, and, at times, to the detriment of other activities in their life. Most circumscribed interests tend to be fairly benign. However, if an individual became interested in, for example, different religious beliefs, espionage or conspiracy theories, it is easy to see the potential for radicalisation.

Despite the lack of strong empirical evidence linking autistic people specifically to terrorist activities, there continues to be a focus upon what are referred to as 'lone actor' terrorist acts. Corner and Gill (2017) and Corner, Gill and Mason (2016) explored this topic and acknowledged that, as previously mentioned in this chapter, it is often the media who appear to decide that a perpetrator is autistic, and it is not always clear whether they have a formal diagnosis.

This topic has been the subject of a number of UK initiatives (e.g. Chisholm and Coulter 2017). However, a study by Walter *et al.* (2021) was the first to specifically examine factors that may predispose autistic persons to be drawn towards radical influences. Their study involved conducting interviews with autistic young people who had been approached by radical groups or who had been identified as being potentially vulnerable to radicalisation. Professionals who had been involved with the young people were also interviewed and included academics, police officers, local authority and education representatives, psychiatrists, psychologists and a specialist nurse.

Walter *et al.*'s findings identified the following 'themes' that were felt to have the potential to increase vulnerability:

1. Difficulties understanding and interpreting interpersonal relationships. These included:
    a. Judging appropriate behaviour (in self and others)
    b. Struggling to work out someone else's intentions (including when being manipulated or 'used' by others)
2. Executive function difficulties:
    a. Challenges in anticipating possible consequences for actions
    b. Difficulty in inhibiting impulses
3. Rigidity of thought – interpreting something as a 'fact' and struggling to shift from this viewpoint.
4. A need for structure: This can make individuals become drawn to organisations that offer a military style structure, particularly cultural, religious or extreme right-wing organisations which often have strict rules and a clear hierarchical structure.
5. Ideologies that align with a person's special interests.

The study also highlighted the potential attraction of online inter-actions for individuals who may find face-to-face socialisation more challenging. Some online communities offer a sense of belonging (this can include being in a space where in-depth knowledge of a particular topic is admired and celebrated). However, this brings with it a risk of young people being exposed to individuals who may be predatory and attempting to 'groom' them.

The issue of the plethora of information that is online about an infinite number of topics was also raised, with a suggestion that some autistic young people may have difficulty in working out what is accurate and truthful.

The context of the young person's family situation was also identified as a potential area of risk. Parents and carers were reported to find it challenging to work out when a special interest in a topic and the known 'quirks' of their children became something more sinister. It was reported that there had been occasions where the potential seriousness of radicalisation was initially overlooked.

Social class and the young person's family background was also identified as a risk factor, with the small number of autistic young people who professionals were aware had become involved in radicalised activity often coming from neglected or 'troubled' backgrounds. At times this was coupled with extreme ideas being passed down as part of their family narrative.

Bullying and being marginalised and excluded by peers was cited by the professionals involved in the research as making autistic young people more susceptible to exploitation.

The paper concluded that there was an urgent need for more training about autism for professionals, particularly those who were responsible for making safeguarding referrals, as it was highlighted that the number of referrals received may be as a result of professionals erring on the side of caution rather than reflecting a genuine increased risk.

The authors also noted that whilst their study largely mirrored the findings of Al-Attar (2020), it was also important to be aware of the young person's family background, their usual behaviour patterns and whether they had been bullied and/or marginalised by peers.

My own experience of working in forensic autism services would suggest that it is also important to evaluate the individual's ability to move on from perceived injustice and their propensity to hold grudges.

The need for a tailored, individualised assessment of risk is undeniable.

Sexual vulnerability and autism

Wider studies into child sexual exploitation do not tend to identify autism specifically or neurodiversity generally as a risk factor for sexual exploitation. However, a paper by Bargiela, Steward and Mandy (2016) explored the experiences of late diagnosed autistic women and high-lighted that many of the women they interviewed for the study reported experiences of victimisation, and their accounts often included reports of passivity and a lack of assertiveness and confidence. One participant described her need to 'please, appease and apologise – do what you're told' (p.3287) in order to feel accepted and receive attention and affection. Another, when describing her initial response to (unwanted) requests for sex, stated that she felt 'pressured' by societal expectations. Amongst this sample, there was a high incidence of reporting of sexual abuse of some kind (64%) with many women reporting feeling 'obliged' or 'pestered' into sexual relations. One young person was groomed by a peer at the bidding of an older man. Another reported finding it difficult to 'read' the intentions of men who were taking an interest in her. Others cited previous experiences of having been rejected as contributing to their vulnerability.

A further important factor which was raised was around uncertainty about their right to say no if they did not want to engage sexually. Some young women did not realise that they could say no, and if they did, they reported that they did not know how.

It is possible that girls who are socially isolated, and who may have missed out on the kind of conversations that their neurotypical peers might have had about sex, may need specific support and guidance around sex and consent. This may be particularly pertinent for those girls who are home-schooled, as they are even more unlikely to have had the opportunity to learn from their peers.

The story of 'Claire' (cited in Eaton 2017, p.185) highlights quite graphically the risks that young autistic women face. Claire went to live alone in London at the age of 19. Having only been in the city for a couple of weeks she found herself lost and alone, and with no charge on her mobile phone. A young man asked her if she was all right and persuaded her to come into his flat, saying he would call her a taxi. She was subsequently imprisoned, raped and threatened with death and pressurised into taking drugs. Claire only managed to escape by pushing her captor down the stairs and running out into the street. This situation was incredibly traumatising for her and had a huge impact upon her mental health, resulting in her being sectioned under the Mental Health Act. She reported that the rape trial was almost as bad as the attack itself. She now acknowledges that she has always had difficulty 'reading' the intentions of others.

A further paper by Mademtzi *et al.* in 2018 carried out interviews with parents of autistic girls with a mean age of 15 years 9 months and explored areas of concern with regard to the potential vulnerability of autistic girls. They expressed particular worries about the pornographic material available on the internet and how confusing these images, and the misleading narrative where this type of behaviour appears to be normalised, would be for their daughters. This echoed the findings of other studies (Cridland *et al.* 2014; Stokes and Kaur 2005). The Cridland *et al.* study reported a case study of an autistic mother (who was being interviewed about the experiences of her autistic daughter) who described having herself slept with lots of boys when she was younger because they told her they 'loved' her (p.9). This mother expressed concerns about her own daughter potentially following the same pattern, describing her as trusting people implicitly.

Aside from sexual vulnerability they also reported that they worried about their daughters' understanding of menstruation, puberty and birth control and the risk of unwanted pregnancy when (and if) they became sexually active. The parents all agreed that they would need to have fairly specific and detailed conversations about consent because talking in ambiguous or abstract terms would be unlikely to be successful. They also reported acknowledging the need to be 'hands-on' parents for much longer than they thought they would have to be, in order to protect their daughters.

A study by Mandell *et al.* (2005) explored the risk of abuse (including sexual abuse) amongst autistic children and found that one in six of their community sample reported some form of sexual abuse.

Examples of exploitation highlight the vulnerability of autistic young people and more particularly those who have either not been diagnosed, are undiagnosed or have been deemed as 'too complex' to work with by professionals. These examples also highlight the need for awareness training amongst professional groups (solicitors, judges and others involved in the criminal justice system).

When an autistic person becomes involved in the CJS

A paper by Blackmore *et al.* (2022) investigated the prevalence rates of those diagnosed as autistic becoming involved in the CJS. They concluded that, although there has been quite limited investigation of this, it is possible that there may be a slightly increased risk of this. The researchers carried out a retrospective review of over 1500 adults (aged between 17 and 75) who were referred to a specialist service for an autism assessment over a 17-year period (2003 to 2020). They found that 23 per cent of their sample had had contact with the CJS. Being male and being diagnosed with comorbid ADHD or a psychotic disorder increased this potential risk. However, the group did not have a comparative group of non-autistic individuals, so it was not possible to determine how this figure compares with the general population.

King and Murphy (2014), in a previous systematic review of the available literature at the time, considered two main types of study: first, those that looked at the prevalence rates of autistic persons who had contact with the CJS, and second, the types of offence committed and any comorbid conditions. They also examined whether there were any particular characteristics amongst an autistic population that would be likely to predispose them to commit certain types of offence. They concluded that autistic persons did not appear to be disproportionately represented in the CJS, or that there were particular crimes that they would be likely to commit. They further concluded, however, that because of the difficulty in accurately establishing the presence (or otherwise) of comorbid mental health difficulties outside of formal mental health settings, it was impossible to speculate about the impact of such comorbidities.

In the course of my clinical career, I have worked in secure forensic inpatient services and have been asked on several occasions to carry out, with colleagues, an assessment for autism of individuals detained in prison. The patients in inpatient services were either detained under

Section 3 of the Mental Health Act or were individuals who had been diverted from the prison system on a Section 37/41 of the Mental Health Act. Those in prison tended to be on an indeterminate sentence of Imprisonment for Public Protection (IPP). IPPs were created by the Criminal Justice Act of 2003 and began being used in 2005. They were designed to protect the public from serious offenders who were not deemed to merit a life sentence. However, offenders were given a minimum 'tariff' or period of time during which they would be detained. Most of the individuals I have been asked to assess were what are referred to as 'post-tariff'. In other words, they had served their minimum sentence, but for these individuals doubt remained as to whether they were sufficiently rehabilitated to be safely released back into the community. Whilst detained, prisoners are expected to complete certain courses that aim to help the individual to understand their behaviour and develop empathy for their victims. These are often standardised 'packages'. The prisoners I have been asked to assess have often failed to demonstrate sufficient (if any) progress on these courses. The offences they have committed have ranged from arson, through to murder and sexual offences. In all cases someone, at some point, has raised the question of whether the individual might be autistic and an assessment is commissioned, very often to inform a Parole Board hearing. Frequently, when the assessment takes place and access is given to the prisoner's file, these individuals will have been referred to as 'complex' or 'difficult' and there is usually a plethora of evidence of them failing to make progress in courses, of misunderstanding or misinterpreting what is said to them, an apparent lack of empathy for their victims, and evidence of rigid thinking around concepts and routines.

Very often, seeing the individual's crime through the lens of an autism diagnosis sheds light on the reasons why they may have 'failed' to make rehabilitative progress.

Sexual offending and autism: prevalence, risk and treatment options

A paper by Mogavero (2016) investigated the prevalence of sexual offending amongst an autistic population and examined incidents of inappropriate approaches to people, exposure of genitals/public masturbation, inappropriate touching and downloading child pornography. It was concluded that although the evidence for criminal behaviour amongst autistic people generally was not strong (Mouridsen 2012; Scragg and Shah 1994), there has been more recent, and growing, concern about an association between autism and sexual offences (Higgs and Carter 2015). Lindsay *et al.* (2014) reported that, compared to a neurotypical population, autistic individuals were reported to commit higher rates (8.5 versus 2.8%) of stalking or non-contact sexual offences.

Paedophilia or autistic misunderstanding?

A paper by Aral, Say and Usta (2018) highlighted the issues faced by a team of clinicians who were asked to assess a 15-year-old girl who had been found to be storing child pornographic images on her computer and subsequently sharing them on social media. The girl had not been previously assessed for autism but had a long history of obsessive interests, frequent internet searches and a lack of friends. The team was asked to assess her for autism and to determine whether she was criminally responsible for her actions.

The background to the case was reported as her having been 'chatting' on a social media platform with an unknown person. This person had developed a fake account and had initiated a conversation with the girl about 'naked people'. He then asked her to send him pictures of naked people, and the girl was reported to have done this without question. She accessed these by searching online and then forwarding the pictures to this individual. When questioned about it subsequently, she struggled to understand why these pictures were not legal as they had been so easily accessible on the internet.

During the course of their assessment, the assessing team established that she was autistic and that she had a long history of obsessive, circumscribed interests which she pursued by researching and collecting information. On this basis, it was decided that she did not fully understand the implications of this type of behaviour and was not, therefore, criminally responsible. It was agreed that she had a poor understanding of social norms and was, therefore, vulnerable to exploitation.

Consequently the issue for the CJS in cases like these is to establish, wherever possible, the underlying motivation behind offences of this kind and attempt to distinguish autistic misunderstanding from sexual deviance.

Paedophilia, paraphilia and autism

The DSM-5 describes paedophilia as recurrent, intense and sexually arousing fantasies, sexual urges and behaviour involving sexual activity with a pre-pubescent child (generally aged 13 years or younger). For a diagnosis of paedophilia, the individual needs to have either acted upon these urges or experienced marked distress and interpersonal difficulties as a result of these urges. The individual needs to be at least 16 years of age and at least five years older than the child(ren) involved. This again raises the issue of vulnerability. In the course of my clinical work, I have come across predominantly young men who have been convicted of offences against a girl under the age of 16 and consequently have found themselves on a sex offenders' register. In some cases, the young men have argued that they did not realise that the girl was underage. This raises the question of whether, and to what extent, autistic young people take into account the usual cues regarding someone's age and how proficient they are at judging someone's age. A paper published by Hobson (1987) examined the ability of autistic children to recognise age- and sex-related characteristics of people. His study showed that some autistic children were significantly less skilled at distinguishing between drawings of a man, a woman, a girl and a boy. It was speculated in this case that they may have paid less attention to both the facial features and the additional cues (clothing, props, etc.) that were provided, which should have indicated age. However, it was likely that many of these children had some degree of intellectual disability. A search of the available literature did not reveal any similar studies that had been carried out on children without intellectual impairment, or any studies that examined this ability in autistic adults, so it is difficult to draw any firm conclusions in this respect.

Paraphilia is described in the DSM-5 as recurrent, intense and sexually arousing fantasy, urge or behaviour that occurs over a period of at least six months and causes significant distress or impairment in sexual functioning.

Kolta and Rossi (2018) highlighted the lack of reported evidence regarding the frequency of paraphilias in an autistic population. Their case study details the history of a young (18-year-old) man who was experiencing suicidal ideation and who had made plans to hang himself. He reported a number of sexual fantasies, one of which involved furry, anthropomorphic animal characters and another involving having sex with a girl and later cutting off her head. The young man was deeply upset by the second fantasy and experienced extreme guilt and shame.

A study by Fernandes *et al.* (2016) concluded that some 10 per cent of higher functioning autistic individuals demonstrated some inappropriate sexual behaviour, and 24 per cent had experienced paraphilic sexual fantasies or classic features of paedophilia, voyeurism or sadomasochism. This may at first glance appear concerning. However, there are two issues to consider here. First, it was clear within the literature that not all these individuals had acted upon these fantasies or were presenting a risk to others. Second, it is not clear how this statistic compares with the number of non-autistic individuals experiencing these types of thoughts or, indeed, how many act upon these.

I was reminded of cases I came across during my time working in adult forensic services with young autistic males. One had a long history of discussing, quite openly, his attraction to young boys and what he would like to do if he was ever in a position to act upon his thoughts. Another disclosed unusual sexual fantasies involving babies and children's cartoon characters. However, neither of these young men had ever acted upon these fantasies and were detained under the Mental Health Act for other reasons. I recall many team discussions when evaluating the potential risk that these two young men could pose to small children when out on leave. It did give me cause to speculate about whether many people have fantasies, but generally would tend to keep them to themselves and not share openly and freely with others. It was argued that, maybe, this was a manifestation of poor social skills and a failure to appreciate the impact upon others of discussing things that some people may find disturbing or unusual, rather like the girl mentioned previously who simply did not realise that the distribution of naked pictures of children was illegal.

The above cases highlight the need for autistic individuals to be understood and supported by those within the CJS.

Legal professionals' understanding of autism

A study by Maras *et al.* (2017) used online surveys to sample the views of legal professionals (judges, barristers and solicitors) regarding their experience of engaging with autistic persons in the criminal courts across England and Wales in the United Kingdom. This study highlighted the need for professionals working within the court system to have an understanding of some of the issues facing autistic defendants and the reasonable adjustments that may need to be made in order to ensure a fair trial.

There have been a number of initiatives designed to ensure that vulnerable individuals, including those who are autistic, have the best possible opportunity to give evidence to the court. One such initiative was the introduction of the Witness Intermediary Scheme, which has proved a positive step (Plotnikoff and Woolfson 2015).

When solicitors and barristers were questioned, they cited 'time out' in court and monitoring the way in which language was used with autistic individuals as the key elements they were aware of in terms of reasonable adjustments. Over half of those questioned stated that, despite preparation and training, they had found cross-examining an autistic individual 'challenging'. When rating their knowledge of autism overall, 75 per cent of respondents reported that they had 'good' knowledge of autism, but only 31 per cent had received formal training. Of those who had received some form of training, it was not clear what type of training they had received, or in what depth the topic had been covered. Worryingly, some of those questioned reported that, at times, they had not even been made aware of the defendant's diagnosis until the trial started.

Members of the autistic community (n = 28) were also questioned about their experience of having been a defendant in court. Results from this revealed that few had received any special consideration. Twenty-five per cent were offered a screen around the witness box, 11 per cent were able to give their evidence via video link and 7 per cent reported that they had been allowed to request that the professionals remove their wigs and gowns. Again, rather worryingly it was noted that only 67 per cent of those individuals questioned had a solicitor present, and only one defendant was offered a meeting with the Crown Prosecution Service (the main agency for the prosecution of criminal cases in the United Kingdom). Several highlighted the lack of awareness of the challenges autistic people can face when asked to provide a verbal narrative, or the memory challenges that some experience. Overall, the study found that, on balance, those questioned felt that they had experienced a lack of understanding of autism from court professionals, and the autistic perception was that any knowledge of autism that professionals had was quite superficial.

This study demonstrates that there was a clear difference between what the legal professionals felt they knew, the steps they felt able to take to support autistic individuals and the way in which this support was experienced by the individuals themselves.

There were also significant concerns about how autistic individuals are perceived in terms of sentencing. Berryessa (2016) carried out a study on the attitude of California High Court judges regarding sentencing autistic offenders. Fifteen of the judges questioned stated that an individual's diagnosis was an important factor in terms of sentencing. However, three of them also stated that knowing that a person was autistic might lead to assumptions being made about that person's impulse control and, consequently, the risk they could potentially pose to themselves and others.

This point brings me back to thinking about the young men I encountered during my time working in forensic services. These young men were detained under the Mental Health Act on a Section 3. Fundamentally, this could mean that they could be detained indefinitely if it was decided that their perceived risk had not decreased, in a similar way to those individuals in prison on indeterminate sentences, who were often also detained long after their original 'tariff'. This raises the question of how to evaluate risk in autistic individuals. Many fail to make adequate 'progress' in traditional prison or inpatient programmes, which are designed to educate or rehabilitate.

Risk assessment in autistic individuals

Shine and Cooper-Evans (2016) acknowledged the particular challenge of evaluating risk and formulating treatment and management plans for autistic individuals in forensic and secure settings.

They reported that between the mid-1990s and 2016, there was a move within forensic services towards the use of structured professional judgement tools (SPJs) within both prison and mental health settings. Examples of the more commonly used tools include the Historical-Clinical-Risk Management-20 (HCR-20; Douglas *et al.* 2014) and the Violence Risk Scale (VRS; Långström *et al.* 2009). However, they noted that these tools have not proved to be especially helpful, or reliable, when working with an autistic population, due to the wide-ranging and varied challenges they can experience, alongside the high level of comorbid conditions and mental health difficulties. Murphy in 2013 had already highlighted that some of the factors examined by the HCR-20 were of questionable use when evaluating the specific risks of autistic offenders. Evaluation of current and future risk is essentially a hypothesis about the various factors that may contribute towards individual risk. Shine and Cooper-Evans, therefore, proposed a framework that could be used to guide clinicians when evaluating risk factors for autistic individuals.

They advocate using what they refer to as 'offence paralleling behaviour' (OPB) as a starting point for a risk assessment. This involves those working with the individual examining their behaviour within the forensic setting and evaluating whether this serves the same function as the behaviour that led to their offence. In other words, is there evidence of a pattern of a particular kind of action, obsession or coping strategy?

A document published by the Royal College of Psychiatrists (2014) identified a number of factors that may need to be considered for autistic individuals in a legal setting. These include the following:

1. Misinterpretation of social relationships
2. Limited emotional awareness
3. Misinterpretation of social rules
4. Difficulties 'reading' social signals
5. Possible difficulty in judging the age of others

6. Vulnerability to exploitation
7. Impulsivity (particularly in combination with comorbid ADHD)
8. Limited appreciation of consequences
9. Overriding preoccupations (which can raise the risk of offences such as stalking)

In addition, they identified factors such as 'incautious frankness' and 'over disclosure', which mirror the examples given earlier in this chapter.

Based upon this document and drawing upon their own experience of working in secure settings, Shine and Cooper-Evans (2016) drew up a list of four factors to consider when evaluating the risk of autistic individuals committing further offences. These were as follows:

1. Pursuit of circumscribed interests/obsessions. These were not deemed to be concerning in isolation. However, risk was deemed to be increased if the individual has become obsessed by a particular person or becomes radicalised as a result of naivety or a desire to 'fit in' with peers.
2. Any identified deficits in theory of mind which may lead to impaired problem solving or social interaction difficulties.
3. Sensory-seeking behaviour, or avoidance of certain sensations.
4. Degree of distress around disruption to rules, or changes in routine.

Shine and Cooper-Evans propose that the use of this framework can support clinicians to formulate risk in autistic persons and put together more effective treatment plans. The framework they have developed pulls together information from the individual's past and the extent to which the four elements above impact upon that person and their like-lihood of reoffending. Although this model has not yet been empirically validated, it does appear to represent a positive step on the part of those working within forensic services in terms of developing autism-specific tools that should allow for a more targeted response and clinical formulation.

Treatment options

A different study (Esan *et al.* 2014) was carried out in a single forensic inpatient service, as the authors had concluded that there was very limited research evidence available that focused upon inpatients with a diagnosis of autism, specifically with regard to treatment options and outcomes.

The study followed the treatment progress of 36 male and six autistic females over a six-year period. It found that the individuals studied presented with a wide range of comorbid conditions and diagnoses, including schizophrenia, epilepsy and personality disorder. These comorbidities meant that initially the focus had tended to be upon pharmacological stabilisation rather than psychological therapy. The majority of these patients were also self-harming.

The authors concluded, somewhat disappointingly, that despite several major reports into autism and offending behaviour (Birmingham City Council 2011; NAS 2011; Scottish Executive Social Research 2004) none gave much emphasis to the type of therapeutic approach that might be helpful. Most of the interventions that were mentioned tended to be more directed towards those individuals with an intellectual disability. This is somewhat concerning given that it is now known that a high percentage of autistic persons do not have an intellectual disability.

Thankfully, a search of the more recent literature did identify one study by Faccini and Allely which was published in 2021 (Faccini and Allely 2021) which discussed the need for a trauma-informed approach to working with autistic individuals in forensic settings.

The authors had highlighted the need to screen for, and identify, traumatic experiences in autistic individuals in a previously published paper (Allely and Faccini 2019). They suggest that routine screening for trauma should be adopted as good clinical practice when working with any autistic person. Many of the difficulties, which could be trauma related, are often attributed to the individual being autistic, and any psychological formulation may fail to consider possible trauma. This can (and does) result in individuals being placed in seclusion or restrained, which could lead to further activation of their trauma response. This is then presumed to be 'dangerous', 'disruptive' or 'attention-seeking' behaviour.

Trauma therapy may need to be modified for autistic persons.

Explanations about the nature of trauma and the trauma response may need to be carefully considered, and care must be taken to ensure that any such explanations are understood.

Several adapted specialist programmes have been developed. These include trauma-informed behavioural interventions (see Harvey 2012) and treatments that utilise EMDR. Kosatka and Ona (2014) investigated the effectiveness of EMDR for a 21-year-old autistic female who had experienced multiple traumas (mainly bullying and physical abuse by her peers). She received therapy three times per week for three weeks (incorporating eight sessions of EMDR therapy). An overall improvement in her trauma symptoms was reported and, perhaps more encouraging, this improvement was maintained at an eight-month follow up. However, it was noted that further large-scale studies were needed before the true efficacy of this type of therapy can be evaluated.

CHAPTER EIGHT

'Perplexing Conditions' and Fabricated and Induced Illness

> This chapter will explore the concept of 'perplexing conditions' in the context of an FII framework. With thanks to Dr Fiona Gullon-Scott, Cathie Long, Andy Bilson and Sally Russell, the other members of the team who prepared the practice guide for the British Association of Social Workers in 2022 (Long *et al.* 2022).

This book as a whole investigates the varied experiences of families where autistic children and young people are deemed to be complex or to present with 'perplexing presentations'. All too often, as will be further covered in the chapter that follows this, a lack of understanding or knowledge about the ways in which autism can present can lead, and has led, to an increasing number of families being accused of having fabricated, exaggerated or simply made up the level of challenge they are experiencing in attempting to secure appropriate support for their children. This chapter will explore the history and legal definition of what is now referred to as fabricated or induced illness.

The history of FII

FII and its predecessor Munchausen Syndrome by Proxy (MSbP) have a chequered history. The term MSbP was initially proposed by Professor Roy Meadow, a paediatrician, in 1977 (Meadow 1977). He used the term to describe a group of 'parents who, by fabrication, have caused them [children] innumerable harmful medical procedures' (Meadow 1982, p.92). In the first instance, Professor Meadow's concern was with young children, stating that: 'Munchausen syndrome by proxy affects children under age 6 years' (Meadow 1982, p.95).

By 1995, Meadow had raised concerns that the diagnosis of MSbP was being overused. He stated that the term MSbP was originally used for 'journalistic reasons' (Meadow 1995, p.534) and said that the criteria he originally proposed 'lacks specificity: many different occurrences fulfil them' (Meadow 1995, p.534).

MSbP, as a formal mental health diagnosis, has not been recognised directly in the *Diagnostic and Statistical Manual of Mental Disorders*. The DSM-5 lists it as 'Factitious Disorder Imposed on Another (FDIoA)'. The defining features that are identified in the DSM-5 include deliberately falsifying either physical or psychological symptoms, either in the person themself or in another. It is acknowledged as a rare phenomenon and requires this deception to be deliberate and without any obvious purpose or reward.

Thus, FDIoA and MSbP both require:

1. that the person *intends* to *deceive*
2. that the behaviour *is not better explained* by another mental disorder.

In the early part of this century MSbP came under wide public scrutiny in the United Kingdom, following several high-profile cases where parents who had been imprisoned for murder had their convictions overturned. In some of these cases Professor Meadow's testimony was strongly criticised for using statistics that exaggerated the likelihood that these parents had killed their children. Following this he was deemed to have given 'erroneous and misleading statistical evidence' (Roberts 2006) and was initially struck off by the British Medical Association, though he was later reinstated at appeal. Ruling on the appeal Mr Justice Collins said that striking him off was unnecessary 'particularly having regard to the fact that he has retired from clinical practice' (cited in Roberts 2006).

Against this background, and further adverse publicity about the use of covert surveillance to identify cases of MSbP, the term fabricated or induced illness was introduced in 2002 with the publication of guidance by the Royal College of Paediatrics and Child Health (RCPCH 2002). The term was used in guidance published in 2008 by the UK Government (HM Government 2008) issued as a supplement to 'Working Together to Safeguard Children' (Social Work England 2020). In 2009, the RCPCH updated their own guidance, and this was reviewed again in 2012 but was not changed. This guidance sought to promote early recognition of FII and broadened the definition saying that the earlier approach focused on 'severe cases where the implication was that the carer was deliberately fabricating or inducing illness in the child' (p.7). In this new broader category, FII was seen to be a spectrum of situations including parents who are 'deliberately fabricating a child's illness; genuinely believes the child to be ill or *is unduly anxious*' (p.7, author's emphasis). This led to the term being used in situations that 'do not involve deliberate fabrication or deception' (p.7).

From this point, it is clear that the guidance around FII has moved away from instances where a parent (or carer) has deliberately caused harm to a child to cases where parents are deemed to be 'unduly anxious' about their children. This inevitably led to parents – who initially reached out for support because they were struggling to support a child with complex challenges – finding themselves under the spotlight when a straightforward reason for their child's difficulties could not easily be identified. Inevitably, this has then led to some parents seeking multiple opinions or assessments.

The current guidance from the RCPCH (updated in March 2021) will influence both medical and social work practice, so a number of key concerns will now be considered in detail, and will include:

- The lack of an evidence base for the extent, progression or treatment of cases.
- Untested alerting signs and no diagnostic tests.
- Definitions which are likely to lead to a large number of children being mistakenly considered as having or being at risk of FII.

The RCPCH (2021, p.6) states that there is 'limited published evidence on prevalence and management of FII'. An evidence-based approach should include research into 'the accuracy and precision of diagnostic tests (including the clinical examination), the power of prognostic markers, and the efficacy and safety of therapeutic, rehabilitative, and preventive regimens' (Sackett 1997, p.3).

What limited research evidence there is tends to focus on MSbP which, because of its rarity, is an exceedingly small and very unrepresentative proportion of cases which are likely to be considered as either a perplexing presentation or FII. A literature review carried out for practice guidelines produced for the British Association of Social Workers (BASW) (Long *et al.* 2022) found no evidence base for the expanded concept of FII; no diagnostic criteria; no research into, or information on, the accuracy or precision of the alerting signs; and no research into the efficacy or safety of the proposed early intervention or treatment proposed. However, it is important to note that there are several reports giving case details of families harmed by being wrongly involved in FII investigations (e.g. Colby 2014; Fiightback 2019; Not Fine in School 2018; Siret 2019), which will be discussed later in this chapter.

The lack of evidence in each of these areas is extremely concerning because it means that:

- Without accurate and precise diagnostic tests there is a high likelihood of providing harmful interventions in cases where children are not being harmed by carers and missing those extremely rare cases where children are being seriously harmed.
- Without research on the prognosis there is no way to accurately identify indicators that children are at risk and the likely course of events including the risk of future harm or to identify cases where there is unlikely to be future harm.
- Without research into the 'efficacy and safety of therapeutic, rehabilitative, and preventive regimens' (Long *et al.* 2022) there is a danger that interventions will harm children and families.

The lack of evidence on prognosis, and the proposed treatment, is illustrated by two of the authors of the RCPCH guidance who in a recent article (Davis, Murtagh and Glaser 2019, p.2) propose this 'early identification' approach but go on to state: 'Whether this can prevent the progression to "full blown" FII remains to be tested.'

Lack of an evidence base for the extent, progression or treatment of cases

What research there is on MSbP does not apply to the wider definition of FII and is itself flawed (for an overview see Eichner 2015, pp.214–218). There are a small number of MSbP cases, as evidenced by case report studies, but these are rare. An international review (Sheridan 2003) found 451 cases published over a 27-year period including duplicate cases; in two thirds of cases there was no independent verification of MSbP; and it embodied the 92 cases in the flawed study, which is discussed below. The RCPCH guidance (RCPCH 2021) itself says there are few recent case studies.

The only epidemiological study on MSbP in the UK was carried out in the early 1990s and covers poisonings, suffocation and cases of MSbP (McClure, Davis and Meadow 1996). It identified an annual rate of children referred to case conferences with a concern about MSbP as 3.8 in every million children aged under 16. The study found that most children were aged under five, and the median age was 20 months. Based mainly on McClure *et al.*'s studies the government's supplementary guidelines state that there is a high mortality rate of between 6 per cent and 10 per cent.

There are severe problems with the McClure research. First, its criteria for MSbP were weak, namely the calling of a child protection case conference. Second, the research looked at poisonings and suffocations of children and failed to distinguish outcomes between poisoning and suffocation not associated with MSbP and MSbP itself. Third, it was carried out by a team including Meadow during the period when over-diagnosis of MSbP led to the miscarriages of justice discussed above.

Correspondence with Peter Sidebotham (who serves on the government Child Safeguarding Practice Review Panel) confirmed that the overviews of serious case reviews in the last 11 years have not identified any deaths directly due to FII. This challenges the research and its view that there is a high level of deaths due to MSbP. This is important because concerns about deaths expressed in the RCPCH guidelines must be tempered by knowledge of the likelihood and even question marks about their occurrence.

Finally, the RCPCH definition of FII covers a wide range of situations from anxiety or disagreeing with medical opinion through to the exceedingly rare deception by fabricating false reports, interfering with samples or illness induction. The guidance (2021, p.17) says 'there is no evidence about the likelihood or factors associated with a parent moving from one point on this continuum to another'. In fact, there is no evidence that these different situations are in any way connected. However, the RCPCH guidance unhelpfully quotes studies of MSbP as if they apply to this wide range of different situations. Despite the use of the term FII, for almost 20 years there is no evidence for diagnosis, prognosis, the proposed treatments or even for the range of situations covered by the definition being in any way connected.

Untested alerting signs and lack of diagnostic criteria

In order to explore this further, it is helpful to refer to the NICE and the RCPCH guidance issued to explain when it may be appropriate to suspect FII.

The NICE Guidelines state the following. Those indicators which could present a potential risk to parents of children with 'perplexing presentations' are highlighted in italics.

Clinicians should suspect that illness may be fabricated or induced if the history, the physical or psychological presentation of the child and any findings of investigations or assessments do not match a recognised clinical picture and, in addition, one or more of the features below are present:

- *Any of the symptoms noted are only observed in the presence of the parent or carer.*
- *Any issues or problems are only seen by the parent or carer.*
- The child demonstrates a poor response to any medication that is prescribed.

- The parent or carer begins to report new symptoms once the previously reported symptoms are resolved.
- The parent or carer reports biologically unlikely symptoms (for example they may reports significant blood loss but the child is not visibly unwell or anaemic).
- *Despite having undergone assessment, and a definite clinical outcome having been agreed, the parent/carer continues to dispute the outcome and seeks further investigations.*

Fabricated or induced illness is a likely explanation even if the child has a past or concurrent physical or psychological condition. (NICE 2017, pp.20–21)

Guidance around FII varies depending upon geographical area within the United Kingdom.

Indicators used in the guidance in Wales (Welsh Assembly Government 2008) include the following. Again, those which could present a potential risk to parents of children with 'perplexing presentations' are highlighted in italics.

- Intentionally attempting to induce symptoms of illness by giving someone medication or other substances (including non-accidental poisoning), or by deliberately attempting to suffocate someone.
- Interfering with genuine medical treatments by deliberately giving an overdose or not giving prescribed medication. It also includes interference with medical equipment, such as drips.
- Claiming that the child has symptoms which are impossible to confirm unless directly seen, for example pain, unexplained vomiting, or fits, particularly if this results in investigation or treatment that later proves to have been unnecessary.
- *Over-exaggeration of presenting symptoms, especially if this results in unnecessary treatment or investigation.*
- Deliberately falsifying medical charts.
- Seeking specialist equipment or treatment that is not needed.
- *Claiming that a child is experiencing psychological stress.*

The RCPCH guidelines proposed a list of 20 alerting signs for fabricated or induced illness. However, they acknowledge there is no research base for this. The guidance says that alerting signs 'are not evidence of FII' (2021, p.18) and that 'A single alerting sign by itself is unlikely to indicate possible fabrication. Paediatricians must look at the overall picture which includes the number and severity of alerting signs' (p.18). It gives no guidance on how to weigh these alerting signs or how to assess their severity. It also does not provide any diagnostic criteria for FII.

The RCPCH Alerting Signs are as follows (again highlighted to illustrate those which are particularly relevant to parents of children with 'perplexing presentations').

In the child

- *The reported symptoms are not seen in the context they are reported in.*
- The child has unusual results from investigations (unusual infections or biological anomalies).
- Unexpected response to prescribed medication.
- Symptoms that are physiologically unlikely or impossible.
- *The child is not attending school or social events.*

In the parent

- *When parents insist upon clinicians continuing to investigate reported difficulties when symptoms cannot be explained by any known condition.*
- *When results of other tests or investigations have failed to provide an explanation for the child's difficulties, and parents still seek further tests and assessment.*
- Constantly reporting new symptoms.
- Frequent attendance at GP's surgery or emergency department.
- *Repeatedly seeking new medical opinions.*
- Parents providing reports for consideration that have been carried out overseas and do not align with UK medical practice.

- *Frequently cancelling appointments.*
- *Parents not able to accept advice and reassurance, seeking further referrals and requesting investigations they have sourced from the internet.*
- *Not allowing professionals to talk to each other.*
- *Making frequent complaints about professionals.*
- Refusing to allow the child to be seen on their own.
- *Answering on behalf of the child, or the child looking to the parent to answer for them.*
- *Repeated changes in school setting (including a switch to home-schooling); changing GP or paediatrician.*
- Factual discrepancies in information about the child's symptoms.
- Parent pushing for life-changing treatment where the clinical need is disputed.

All of the items in italics are those areas where parents of children presenting with complex or 'perplexing' presentations are particularly vulnerable. In many instances, the difficulties, or behavioural challenges, that the child or young person experiences are only seen by the parents in the family home. The child or young person may 'mask' or 'camouflage' their difficulties, only revealing the true extent of their distress in the safety of their own home, with people they feel able to trust.

These criteria can also present a huge risk for parents seeking recognition of the PDA profile, seen in some autistic children and young people. Because of the huge controversy that still surrounds this description of behaviour, many NHS trusts either do not recognise this profile, or actively reject any discussion of it as a possible explanation for a child or young person's difficulties, and many parents feel – quite justifiably – anxious, upset and angry when they do not feel heard or have their concerns about their children taken seriously. This may well lead them to seek multiple opinions, or request further investigation of their child's difficulties, or challenge professional opinion. In addition, many children with complex presentations are unable to attend school and are home-schooled, and discussions about 'social exclusion' or limited access to social activities is very subjective and will largely be determined by the child or young person's own preferences in this area.

Consequently, using the alerting signs to identify FII and PP has major drawbacks, which are likely to lead to high levels of over-identification, and consequent harm to children and families, for the reasons stated above. First, the vagueness of the signs that require a subjective determination by medical staff (e.g. 'not able to accept reassurance', 'vexatious complaints' and 'inappropriately seeking multiple medical opinions'). Second, they also fail to take into account the differences between parents of children where illness is indeed fabricated and the situation of caring parents who are dealing with children who have uncommon presentations of diagnosed conditions.

There is a distinct lack of epidemiological research on the incidence of FII (RCPCH 2021) and no official figures for the number of investigations and subsequent findings of FII. However, several sources suggest a large rise in parents being investigated for fabricating or inducing illness in their children. Davis *et al.* (2019) state that paediatricians in larger hospitals have reported upwards of 50 cases under investigation, and there is growing evidence that many of these investigations are unnecessary (Colby 2014) and seriously harm families and children (Siret 2019). This is reflected in news reports and statements by organisations representing sufferers of a range of diseases and disabilities (e.g. Autism Eye 2018; Ehlers-Danlos Society n.d.; Siret 2019) or difficulties (e.g. Not Fine in School 2018). Parents who have undergone investigation report that they have faced bullying and forms of state oppression, such as being threatened with having their children removed from the family and subjected to enforced rehabilitation (typically in a psychiatric unit) or having their children placed on the 'At Risk register'.

The over-identification of risk in this difficult area is thus a key issue which this chapter seeks to highlight. It is essential for social work practitioners, and other professionals, to work together to ensure that all children are effectively protected from the exceedingly rare situations in which parents cause their child to be significantly harmed, by falsifying medical signs or causing them to have unnecessary and invasive medical treatment.

However, it is equally important to protect children from the harm done to them, their parents/caregivers and their families when they are wrongfully investigated in relation to suspicions of FII (e.g. see

Fiightback 2019; Siret 2019). These impacts can be enormous and long lasting. Many parents have consistently reported a stigma associated with FII where historical accounts remain on their medical records resulting in long-term discrimination, even where the original concerns were unfounded. It is thus important to have clear guidance to help make effective judgements about cases of concern.

At the time of writing, the 2008 guidance remains in force in England, though the Department for Education (DfE) is considering withdrawing it. The English guidance (DCSF 2008) says terminology in this area has been under debate. Therefore, to ensure a focus on the welfare of the child, it refers to FII rather than using a particular term. It stipulates that the guidance is for children where there is concern that they are suffering significant harm, and primarily focuses on physical abuse caused by FII (p.8) and is supported in Working Together to Safeguard Children (Social Work England 2020, p.103). A more appropriate definition would be to focus on the (extremely rare) situations where the parent or carer is actively involved in fabricating the child's medical history, tampering with records or medical tests, or is inducing illness. The RCPCH itself recognises the lack of an evidence base for their proposed approach, stating: 'In the absence of published evidence, we relied on extensive consultation and expert consensus' (2021, p.6). Given this lack of an evidence base and the need for consensus, it is notable that in the list of consultees who 'agreed to be listed' (p.6), there is a total absence of organisations representing key safeguarding bodies including social work, education and the police. This is particularly concerning as the guidance focuses on safeguarding issues and guidelines for making EHCPs.

In conclusion, the new guidance departs from a focus on serious harm caused by carers who deliberately fabricate or induce illness and uses unresearched and untested alerting signs to attempt to identify cases early. The guidance also appears to exaggerate the likely harm caused by a wide group of unrelated situations, including by parents who are anxious about their child's health. At the same time, there is no recognition within the guidance of the potential harm caused by wrongful identification of cases and the damage to children and families caused by this.

Over the past few years, several voluntary organisations (Not Fine in School and Fiightback) in the United Kingdom have been set up to support parents who have been accused of FII and are currently fighting for a Parliamentary review of the situation.

The Parent and Carer Alliance (PCA) (2019) surveyed a number of parents who were sharing their experiences of having been accused of FII online. These experiences were shared, without prompting, and presented a consistent and repeated picture of frustration when trying to access support for their children, not being listened to and of being accused of poor parenting.

Ultimately, the PCA gained permission to share the experiences of 12 families who all had dealings with one English local authority. These parents highlighted the challenges of supporting children with additional needs, extremely challenging behaviour and complex, or 'perplexing', presentations, which are not always straightforward to assess, diagnose or support. Parents reported that when these challenges were further compounded by accusations of poor parenting, the long-term impact was described as 'profound and long-lasting' (PCA 2019, p.1).

The author of this report received no payment for it and had over 30 years' experience of working as a qualified social worker, including working in safeguarding and child protection services. In 11 out of the 12 cases the accusations were found to be unsubstantiated, and child protection services were not instigated.

The majority of the parents impacted by this felt that the allegations of possible FII had come about as a direct result of either asking for additional support, not being happy with the level or type of support offered, or because they had made a complaint.

The families were subsequently asked to discuss the impact that these accusations had had upon their families. One mother reported that she felt unable to go back to work because of what might be included on her Disclosure and Barring Service check (DBS). A DBS check is carried out in the United Kingdom prior to a person commencing employment with vulnerable children or adults and outlines any past, or current, concerns in this area.

Another common theme was reports of depression, anxiety and a general reluctance to trust services in the future. One mother explained that, often, inaccuracies in children's records go uncorrected, causing further distress. In all cases, anxiety and fear were reported, along with symptoms of PTSD. Others reported financial loss, loss of career and even family breakdown.

In all but one of the cases (where there were other factors at play), there was no eventual benefit to either the child or family and no additional support was offered.

Of particular concern was the issue of a lack of appropriate diagnosis. Ten out of the twelve cases reported noted that allegations of possible FII were made without the child having received an assessment and/or diagnosis. In one case where a diagnosis was made, it was rejected and subsequently disregarded.

The case of the child whose diagnosis was made and subsequently rejected is the most relevant to the topic of this book. The child was eight years old and had a diagnosis of autism with the PDA profile. Strategies suggested for children with this profile of difficulties had proved very effective in the home environment. PDA was not, at that time, 'recognised' by either the child's school or the paediatric team in the family's local area.

The allegation of FII was made after the child's mother attended a meeting at his school. She had requested the meeting in an attempt to get some advice, or support, as her child was experiencing 'meltdowns' and challenging behaviour when he returned home from school. The child's mother was open in admitting that his father was struggling to manage this and was asking if it was possible for school staff and her to work together as she believed that he was 'holding it together' whilst at school and letting his feelings of frustration and anxiety out when he reached the safety and security of his home environment. This presentation is seen very frequently in autistic children and has come to be known as 'masking' or 'camouflaging'. However, instead of supporting the child's mother, she was told that the child's difficulties were due to her own 'mental health problems' (PCA 2019, p.15) and that she was not 'strict enough' (p.17), and it was concluded that, as parents, they were effectively abusing their child.

Children's social care were subsequently contacted. However, no safeguarding procedures were initiated in this case. The child's father was later diagnosed with stress and depression, and the child continued to receive no additional support in school.

Another family who also had an autistic child, and who also found themselves at breaking point, reached out to social care for support. In this case a social care assessment upheld the concerns, and a child protection conference was held. The children were the subject of a child protection plan for three months before being discharged. However, the child's mother remains fearful of any further contact with social services and is reluctant to approach professionals for any issue, behavioural or health-related, in case she faces further accusations, as she is all too aware that this episode remains on her child's file.

The case study below illustrates how quickly a situation, where a mother is concerned about her child's wellbeing, can escalate to child protection proceedings. Fortunately, in this case, the family were able to secure the services of an independent social worker, who was able to put forward a case whereby the child protection concerns were put aside, and the most appropriate support was recommended for him.

DANIEL'S STORY

Daniel is a 14-year-old boy who lives with his mother Jane and his older brother.

Jane reported that, during the pregnancy, it was thought that Daniel might be small for dates, and Jane described herself as very stressed during the pregnancy. Daniel was born at home, at term, and delivered as a healthy baby, except for a Staphylococcal infection which developed at three days old, and resolved, responding well to treatment. Jane described Daniel as quite an active, demanding baby, but that he was easy to settle. She first noticed that there was something different about him around the age of two. He used to cry a lot and become distressed for quite long periods of time. He wouldn't settle into a playgroup and would smear paint on himself rather than the paper. He also became very controlling of Jane, insisting that she perform certain actions in a very specific manner. Jane recalled that he used to love role playing being a mechanic, but it was very difficult to join in his play. At around the age of three, he loved model sharks and sea creatures, but as he got older, he started to become interested in facts and statistics. Jane recalled that he did not use pointing to make requests; she remembers he used to scream, and she didn't know what he wanted.

Daniel was ultimately diagnosed with autism, anxiety, selective mutism, a demand avoidant profile (PDA) and sensory differences.

His anxiety became severe around the transition from Key Stage 1 to Key Stage 2. When a teacher left abruptly, he became very anxious about school. This culminated in an episode where he was physically restrained. This would have been an extremely distressing event for any child, but especially for an autistic child. It resulted in him not being able to leave the house for a period of six months. This resulted in Jane deregistering him from school.

Subsequently, a child and family assessment was initiated by Jane's local authority children's social care following a referral which had raised concerns that Daniel had not had consistent access to a learning environment or social opportunities outside of the family home or with anyone other than his mother. A section 47 enquiry was carried out which concluded that the concerns 'were substantiated but that the children were not at ongoing risk of significant harm'.

The section 47 assessment further recommended that Daniel was to have a child in need plan, which was in place for over 12 months. Children's social care, however, later concluded that as there had been no positive change or progression and his situation had deteriorated, they had ongoing concerns in relation to him remaining unseen by professionals, being socially isolated and not accessing an education other than provided by Jane. Daniel was then made subject to child protection planning under the category of emotional abuse.

It was noted that Daniel had a low distress tolerance and that high levels of distress were triggered by change, or even perceived change. Jane reported that the emergency services had been required to attend on three separate occasions, to support her in managing him. On the first occasion he was temporarily held under S136 of the Mental Health Act, and on the second occasion, he was restrained by four officers and transferred to hospital where he was chemically sedated. On the third occasion, the police officers attending the incident deemed it appropriate to aim tasers at him. She argued that making 'progress' with Daniel was 'not as easy as simply adopting a more robust approach (to managing him)'.

An educational psychologist was commissioned to critically assess Daniel's EHCP and to ascertain if the current education provision at the named school was able to meet his needs. The report affirmed that 'Daniel's Social, Emotional and Mental Health difficulties mean that he is unable to access educational provision within a school setting and that his difficulties needed to be prioritised and addressed by experienced professionals who understood and were trained to work with young people with his level of anxiety and complex needs'. The report also concluded that he was likely to need 'considerable and co-ordinated multi-agency support to move to a position where he is able to re-engage socially and participate in activities outside the home'.

CHAPTER NINE

Social Work Practice, Neurodivergence and Fabricated or Induced Illness

CATHLEEN LONG

This chapter (written by an independent social worker) examines how an investigation of suspected FII should be managed from a social work and legal perspective and includes personal accounts of an autistic mother whose children were removed.

As an independent social worker and expert witness, I assess neurodivergent children and young people with an array of complex needs, providing evidence for the social care components of their EHCPs. I often follow the assessment by giving expert evidence in a Special Educational Needs and Disability Tribunal. I enjoy this aspect of my work because it is very similar to when I worked as a forensic mental health social worker, where I needed to gather and analyse information and make evidence-based decisions about needs and outcomes, writing reports and presenting verbal evidence to the Mental Health Review Tribunal and the Ministry of Justice. Throughout my social work career, I have sought to utilise a person-centred approach whereby my focus is on mindful consideration of the holistic needs of the person I am assessing, but not to the exclusion of their parents and caregivers. I come from the stance 'I'm-OK,

You're-OK' and seek to work collaboratively with individuals rather than perceiving them as 'less-than' me. I wholeheartedly agree that the needs of all children are paramount, and protecting their welfare is vital. However, I also appreciate the harm caused when families are left without support and start to fall to pieces, with the risk of their child or children needing to be accommodated by the flawed and sometimes harmful care system which can fail children, particularly those with complex needs. For example, a young autistic woman I worked with had been placed in 14 different foster care placements within a year, following a succession of placement breakdowns, which does not bode well for an already traumatised child who struggled with change and transitions.

In recent years, I have received numerous enquiries from parents who have been accused of FII, or parents who are fearful that this will happen. Initially, there were a trickle of referrals until last year I had 26 contacts within one week. As a neurodivergent professional who primarily works with neurodivergent people, it is noticeable that a proportion of parents accused of FII are themselves neurodivergent. Some are diagnosed, some self-identify, and others have no awareness of this. Whereas the diagnostic criterion for autism presents a medical model of deficits and treatment, as an autistic professional, I prefer the concept of autism being a 'difference'. Increasingly, more people are being recognised as autistic in later life. There are many factors which have influenced misdiagnosis and missed diagnoses which have already been explained in Chapter Two. Autistic people have a different way of processing information, interpreting social communication and relating to other people. Invariably we also have a different perception of our sensory environment, which is unique from one individual to another.

All too often, professionals believe FII is the same as the historical diagnosis MSbP. This diagnostic terminology has since been replaced with the term factitious disorder imposed on another (FDIoA), which is an extremely rare diagnosis and involves recurrent episodes where a parent/caregiver intends to deceive by falsifying physical or psychological symptoms or induces injury or disease in another person (APA 2013, p.325). The reality is FII is *not* a clinical diagnosis and is *not* included in the DSM-5 (APA 2013). However, this confusion is not at all surprising, as when I recently visited an NHS website, it stated: 'Fabricated or induced illness (FII) is a rare form of child abuse… FII used to be known as "Munchausen's syndrome by proxy"…' (NHS n.d.). FII is described by the RCPCH as:

> a clinical situation in which a child is, or is very likely to be, harmed due to parent(s) behaviour and action, carried out in order to convince doctors that the child's state of physical and/or mental health and neurodevelopment is impaired (or more impaired than is actually the case). (RCPCH 2021, p.11)

The primary motivations cited by the RCPCH as to why parents exaggerate or create their child's difficulties include the psychological needs of the parent, their need for attention (particularly from doctors), their need for their child to be perceived as unwell or disabled, and 'the parent's erroneous beliefs, extreme concern and anxiety about their child's health'. The latter can include 'a mistaken belief that their child needs additional support at school and an Education Health and Care Plan (EHCP)' (p.13). Therefore, parents requesting an EHCP for their child can automatically find themselves in a position where they are accused of FII. I have experiences where parents have enjoyed positive relationships with school staff which have instantaneously changed when they have requested their child is assessed for an EHCP, and/or they have cause to make a complaint. Furthermore, when families have been in crisis and they have self-referred to children's social care, I have heard numerous accounts, particularly from autistic parents, who have been subjected to child protection investigations because professionals instantaneously believe FII is underpinning parental behaviour. In one extreme situation, a child was forcibly removed from their parents' care, and, when the case was presented to court, both parents were accused of FII. In reviewing the documentation, it was apparent the accusations were not evidence based, and the assertions of the clinical commissioning group (CCG) and local authority were themselves fabricated. However, when injustice occurs, there is no clear recourse for parents or their children, who are deeply traumatised and exhibiting symptoms of chronic post-traumatic stress.

As a neurodivergent professional, it is a common experience for me to meet parents of neurodivergent children who are themselves autistic but show no awareness of this. Those who know they are autistic often choose not to disclose this to professionals because of their fear of being judged and discriminated against. Autism is often perceived as a series of 'deficits', which is explicitly supported in the DSM-5. However, many autistic people recognise they are 'different' whilst accepting that being different does not equate to being less-than others. Autistic people often grow up with a sense of feeling different with the conscious and subconscious messages they receive from parents, caregivers and teachers being carried into adulthood and underpinning their beliefs about themselves. An example of this is when an autistic child who struggles to cope in social situations is labelled as 'difficult and awkward' and therefore they learn to adapt their behaviour to fit others' expectations. The implicit message they receive is 'Don't be you', causing them to grow up masking or camouflaging their behaviour. Another message can be 'You're the odd one out, you don't fit in', which can lead to the belief 'I think I don't belong'. All too often, autistic people are told 'You don't look autistic' or 'That's really autistic behaviour', which painfully discounts their lived experience and thus undermines their integrity.

Notably, as an independent social worker, I am aware how often family courts request an assessment of autistic parents using the Parent Assessment Manual Software-4 (PAMS4), which is designed to evaluate the parenting capabilities of parents with a learning difficulty/disability. Without intending to undermine or denigrate this specific assessment, the PAMS4 assessment tools are not designed with an autistic parent in mind. Professionals can unintentionally adopt the misguided notion that being autistic automatically equates to having a learning difficulty/disability. When a professional does not have autism expertise, there is the risk of them imposing a neurotypical approach to parenting, which fails to identify and appreciate the positive qualities and strengths a lot of autistic parents offer. There can be a misconception that autistic people lack empathy, whereas the reality is they can be highly empathic although their style of empathy might be expressed differently.

Autistic parents who have historically experienced difficulties with their mental health, or women with a historical *mis*diagnosis of EUPD, are often subjected to immediate discrimination by services because of this. As a very experienced mental health social worker, I have seen numerous judgements and labels where people with a 'personality disorder' diagnosis are wrongly labelled as 'attention-seeking', 'demanding' and 'making up their problems'. There can be blatant or subliminal assumptions made by professionals that, as well as creating their own difficulties, these parents have a deep-seated need to exaggerate their child's problems as a way of eliciting attention to meet their own emotional needs. A large percentage of autistic women and girls I have worked with have been initially diagnosed with a 'personality disorder', with professionals, including social workers and psychiatrists, choosing to accept the original misdiagnosis rather than understanding or acknowledging that being autistic does not equate to having an emotionally unstable personality disorder. The following is a harrowing account, written by an autistic mother, who expresses the trauma and distress she and her children have experienced because of wrongful allegations of FII. The essence of her experience was how the local authority preferred to attribute her difficulties to a previous diagnosis of EUPD, rather than recognising her as an autistic parent of neurodivergent children:

AN AUTISTIC MOTHER'S STORY

My family's experience was traumatic; the pain can never be expressed in words, nor ever leave us, because we know that at any point until the age of 18 is reached, as an autistic mother of neurodivergent children we can be reaccused repeatedly. The fear of having our children removed never leaves. That there is never justice, there's no accountability and no apology.

How can anyone truly express the guilt, pain, shame, fear, isolation and resulting trauma when you know from reading subject access requests that the events that unfolded did so because you raised concerns about a specialist school not providing provision, when a local authority failed to provide an educational package for years, could not find a suitable educational provision, because you threatened a judicial review, because you asked for support and led to the reactive, aggressive response and false accusation of FII from the local authority?

How that sense/need for justice – that deep-seated desire to give your children a better life, to not have your experiences – drives you to ensure their needs are identified and then met with appropriate support because you want them to have a better life and reach their potential. Unless you had the lived experiences yourself of being failed and unlawfully held in hospitals because of a misdiagnosis, you can never truly appreciate that desire to ensure that history doesn't repeat itself, but unfortunately that is then misconstrued and twisted to mean you are exaggerating the children's needs. How, when you sought assessments from the NHS, they were blocked because your parental diagnosis was used to justify your child's behaviour (lack of boundaries), but then when you go to independent clinicians and needs are identified and recommendations are made, the professionals within the local authority use accusations of FII to hide their failings.

How do you explain to anyone that you ended up safeguarding your family from the ones you've turned to for support? Especially when the rhetoric in training, research and in the media portrays us as problematic, inept, refrigerator mothers with little to no capability for empathy. When there exists a list suggesting that the risk of FII is essentially autism and all co-occurring conditions. We are isolated in our communities, often have little family support, and/or are single parents; many like me meet that tick list used by social services.

Often it would surprise me when I asked professionals about their knowledge of disabilities. They would often admit no knowledge, train-ing or experience but were working within the disability team. How can we truly share the frustration of having to prove our innocence against personal and professional opinions, misrepresentation of facts to police, medical and educational professionals, but be denied the opportunity to do so? Or when subject access requests are withheld, and automatic extensions are applied, which disables you from being able to defend yourself? Or that you haven't got the financial resources to get legal help or support, and are denied counselling and advocacy, for you and your children, who go through this process with you. When you approach regulatory bodies, no one is willing to investigate because of perceived risk from those involved in accusing you. The painful reality is that a criminal is afforded grace of doubt, they must be proven guilty; but for parents like myself, it is the opposite: no evidence is required or it is deemed necessary to levy the accusation of FII. Further, there is the issue of the ways in which the numbers of those accused are hidden, by not actively documenting the accusation of FII, but using other terminology implying abuse and neglect.

For me the most painful memory that even now is hard to address was taking my children to school knowing I may never see them again, scared of what would happen to them knowing the professionals had not prepared the children in any way and instead I had to prepare them for the possibility of being taken from me and reassure them whilst inside my heart was being ripped apart. That pain you cannot describe, and it never leaves. It's as though your heart, body and mind are being ripped into a thousand pieces; you are trying to be calm, trying to hold it together, but inside you're falling apart. The nights crying wishing the ground would swallow you up whole and then getting up. Every email, every letter, every meeting, every visit involves listening to misrepresentations of truth, having the evidence to disprove it, but not being allowed to present it.

Then on that day, by a miracle your children and you are given a chance and you go home together, and you then read the paperwork that no one had seen prior to the family court process. You then dis-cover they have already placed your child for adoption and the other child was going to be put into a foster care placement. Again, you break down in tears, realising not only were you about to lose your children, but they were going to lose each other.

You can never really share with anyone the level of pain experi-enced by your family in these processes, and the sense of failure when you cannot get justice; and the professionals who did this to your family remain working with vulnerable families, and are never held to account, whilst you are left broken, hypervigilant, with no trust in the system. Then, you are held accountable for not trusting those who tried to break up your family. You know also that no one in your community would have cared if your family were broken and your children taken into care, because they too buy into the narratives created portraying us as bad parents, the 'refrigerator mother' created within historical and current guidance very reminiscent of Bettelheim's parentectomy. That knowledge of how vulnerable as a family you will remain, the painful reality that, as a demographic group, we are not afforded the same protection as others. We are already presumed guilty because others have decided that is the case. Our voices and experiences are silenced, the pain buried deep, justice never to be achieved and never an apology to be given. No words can ever adequately express what we went through.

The RCPCH's alerting signs

Considering the above autistic mother's experiences, it is important to re-evaluate the alerting signs presented by the RCPCH. There is a necessity to consider alternative reasons as to why an autistic parent of a child with special educational needs might automatically meet the criteria for FII. The following are listed by the RCPCH specific to parental behaviour and are said to be indicative of FII.

Parents' insistence on continued investigations instead of focusing on symptom alleviation when reported symptoms and signs are not explained by any known medical condition in the child

Sometimes parents' insistence on further investigations are crucial to the wellbeing of their child. Shortly after the birth of my daughter, I noticed subcutaneous lumps on the back of her thighs and on her head. When I questioned this, I was immediately fobbed off by the ward doctor. However, I was persistent, and my daughter was diagnosed with an unusual presentation of Neuroblastoma. A couple of years ago I met another autistic mother who instinctively knew her daughter was unwell; she was vomiting and complaining of stomach pains. Each time she took her daughter to see their general practitioner, she was told there was nothing medically wrong, the child was 'malingering', with the parent being advised to give her pain relief syrup. The mother was subsequently reported to children's social care by the doctor and investigated for FII. It later transpired her daughter had a twisted colon. Aside from physical health conditions, there are many instances where parents have suspected their child is autistic with other presentations related to this, for example ADHD, acute anxiety, PDA, hypermobility syndrome and sensory processing differences. When staff in school do not realise the extent of the child's difficulties because of compliance and masking, parental accounts have been attributed to FII, even when they have pursued an expert diagnosis from credible practitioners.

My experience is that, first and foremost, parents will evaluate 'What am I doing wrong?', thus questioning their parenting approach before considering other options, such as specialist examinations and investigations. One autistic parent wrote:

> Prior to my son being diagnosed as autistic, I changed and adapted my style of parenting in the hope I would find a better way to meet his needs and to reduce incidents of distressing behavioural presentations, where he'd scream, kick, and pull my hair.

It is usually only when all options have been exhausted that a parent will seek to engage expert professionals to assess whether their child is neurodivergent. Typically, this will start with a visit to their general practitioner to initiate a referral to their local CAMHS. However, if this referral is not fruitful, or they are informed there is a two-year wait for an autism diagnostic assessment, parents might opt to engage privately funded experts to assess their child. The reality is that without these expert assessments, they have no other way to ensure the needs of their child are understood before an EHCP can be considered. Many children and young people I work with have a string of interrelated diagnoses, with some of these becoming more apparent when the gap between the child's developmental presentation and that of their peers widens. There might be instances when a parent is determined for their child to be given a specific diagnosis, but this has rarely been my experience.

Repeated reporting of new symptoms

I would be concerned if a parent was reporting extreme symptoms which cannot be verified by others. However, rather than dismissing them, there is a need for each presentation to be investigated before FII is considered. For example, I have worked with parents whose autistic children have manifestations of non-epileptic seizures following episodes of trauma, which medical professionals have disputed. Also, once a parent has recognised their child has difficulties, they may start to notice differences in the child's behaviour, sometimes subtle ones, and together these all form part of the bigger picture. One parent reported:

> When my son was first identified as autistic, I had no awareness that his sensory processing differences caused him to eat a very limited diet and to be intolerant of certain smells and noises. Hence my knowledge and reporting of his difficulties increased as my awareness grew.

Sometimes, parents feel they must repeatedly report new presentations because, unless they do, they do not receive the services and support they need. However, the cumulative effect of persistently reporting concerns can and does lead to investigations into the possibility of FII.

Repeated presentations to and attendance at medical settings including emergency departments

How many times have parents resorted to taking their child to an Accident and Emergency (A&E) department because they have no other option? It is a parent who is desperately concerned about their child's welfare who would keep presenting them at their local hospital. For example, a parent who is very concerned about their autistic teenager, who has self-harmed and is expressing suicidal thoughts, might take them to their local A&E department because CAMHS has not engaged nor offered the child/young person the support they need. Realistically, if a parent was travelling from one A&E department to another in different towns and presenting their child with difficulties which cannot be substantiated nor quantified, this indeed merits further exploration and investigation. Many parents repeatedly take their child to see their general practitioner because their expressions of concern about their child's development and wellbeing are not being proactively listened to, but this is not FII. To reiterate, most often it is a parent who feels desperation and anxiety about their child's wellbeing who will repeatedly access medical services. However, this does not negate that there will be an extremely small percentage of parents who could meet the diagnostic criterion for FDIoA.

Inappropriately seeking multiple medical opinions

When a parent is seeking answers because they intuitively know that their child is physically unwell, or believe they are neurodivergent, they may be required to seek multiple professional opinions to secure sufficient evidence to support the issuing of their child's EHCP. This might be deemed by professionals as 'inappropriate'; however, in today's economic climate, parents have huge hurdles to jump to ensure the education, health and social care needs of their child are properly met. There are also conditions which are disputed amongst medical professionals including myalgic encephalomyelitis/chronic fatigue syndrome (ME/CFS) because there is not a specific diagnostic test. Consequently, people with ME/CFS have been accused of malingering or told their difficulties are psychologically based, rather than any acceptance of their difficulties with cognition and episodes of extreme fatigue. There are also interprofessional disputes about the existence and prevalence of PDA, with some CAMHS teams refusing to accept this as a diagnosis or presentation. A further diagnosis too often disputed is the autoimmune condition paediatric acute-onset neuropsychiatric syndrome/paediatric autoimmune neuropsychiatric disease associated with Strep (PANS/PANDAS). With PANS/PANDAS, 'One day your child is well; over the next week or so they become burdened with conditions such as severe anxiety, OCD [obsessive compulsive disorder], tics, eating disorders or trichotillomania (hair pulling)' (PANDAS/PANS UK 2022).

Providing reports by doctors from abroad which conflict with UK medical practice

I have worked with parents whose children have received lifesaving and pioneering treatment from clinicians outside of the United Kingdom. It has been at great financial cost, particularly because the success of the treatment must be monitored and reviewed once the initial treatment has finished. Parents quickly become experts in their child's condition and are ready to impart their knowledge to UK clinicians to ensure their child continues to receive the best treatment possible. It can be at the point where a parent seeks to re-engage with local NHS doctors that FII becomes an issue. There might be the rare occasion when a parent subjects their child to unorthodox treatments abroad, but I would consider this to be fuelled by desperation and anxiousness on the parents' behalf, rather than attributable to fabrication. Within the UK there are disputes about different approaches to supporting an autistic child including some very strong opposition to applied behaviour analysis (ABA), and parents insisting their autistic child follows a casein-free/ gluten-free diet. These are parental preferences and as professionals we may have our own opinions, but these should not be imposed upon parental preferences unless there is evidence suggesting that a child is being harmed.

Child repeatedly not brought to some appointments, often due to cancellations

Autistic children often experience varying degrees of anxiety which can be exacerbated by changes in their daily routine and the need to meet the expectations of others. Attending an appointment with an unknown professional can cause them anxiety. Sometimes, the expectation of having to get up, get dressed and go out of the house with a parent is far too overwhelming for an autistic child, particularly when they have a demand avoidant presentation. 'Demand avoidance' involves not being able to do certain things at specific times, even enjoyable activities, because high levels of anxiety cause an innate avoidance reaction. High anxiety can lead to an autistic person being unable to speak in different environments. For example, a child I know well could not speak outside of his home, and instead he used facial expressions and eye movements to communicate. He was later diagnosed with acute anxiety and ADHD. Therefore, it is not surprising when a parent/caregiver arrives for an appointment without the child in question because enforcing their attendance can be too arduous and distressing for the child, and parent. When a child does manage to attend their appointment, they might rely upon their parent to speak on their behalf because their anxiety precludes them from contributing.

Not able to accept reassurance or recommended management, and insistence on more, clinically unwarranted, investigations, referrals, and continuation of or new treatments (sometimes based on internet searches)

Many parents I have worked with have realised their child has difficulties significantly earlier than educationalists, medical practitioners and social workers. One of the primary features I have witnessed is when social workers attribute a child's difficulties to a parent being unable to implement and adhere to appropriate boundaries. However, traditional parenting approaches can be futile for an autistic child who is demand avoidant, with professionals trying to impose a neurotypical parenting approach with little understanding of why this doesn't work. A regular outcome following a children's social care assessment is the recommendation for an autistic parent to attend a parenting course. Social workers are generally attuned to a neurotypical parenting approach and can misunderstand that an autistic parent chooses or needs to parent differently. Although the issuing of an EHCP for a child should be dependent on need, as opposed to a formal diagnosis, usually parents must privately fund multiple specialist diagnoses and assessments to evidence their child's special educational needs. To secure an EHCP for a neurodivergent child can involve a succession of diagnostic and specialist assessments, including those of a speech and language therapist, educational and/or clinical psychologist, psychiatrist, occupational therapist, and sometimes an independent social worker.

Additionally, when an autistic child has complex issues, such as disordered eating or gender dysphoria, this can increase the number of specialist assessments needed. For a professional who does not understand the spectrum of co-occurring difficulties an autistic child can experience, gaining expert professional reports can seem like a parent is on a mission to collect diagnoses, when the reality is they want to establish the existence and extent of their child's difficulties for the purpose of achieving the right support. One of the features of many autistic parents is their attention to detail and a need to find solutions to their child's difficulties, leading them to undertake extensive internet searches and masses of exploration until understanding and resolution is achieved.

Objection to communication between professionals

If we consider the power of organisations and the influence they can have over the lives of children with additional needs, it is not surprising that some autistic parents become mistrustful of information shared without their knowledge, particularly when they have numerous hurtful experiences of oppression, discrimination and judgement. I am aware of parents who have accessed their records using a SAR and have consequently been mortified by the conclusions reached by professionals and the inaccuracy of information shared. When we put this into the context, one of the issues for autistic parents is they can have difficulties determining who they can trust and they need to have some control over who is talking about them, or with whom their personal information is being shared. If a parent perceives that a professional is judging them and misunderstanding their child's needs, they are very likely to object to the sharing of information by professionals outside of the child protection arena. For an autistic parent, it can feel tantamount to professional collusion, where those in positions of authority are stacking up evidence to discount their needs and the needs of the child.

Frequent vexatious complaints about professionals

The term 'vexatious' means 'vexing or tending to vex', and within the law, it is the legal action or proceeding 'instituted without sufficient grounds...to cause annoyance or embarrassment to the defendant' (Collins Dictionary, 2022). However, I know from my extensive experience as a social worker that the parent/caregiver or family member who repeatedly complains because they are not being listened to, or their needs are being repeatedly disregarded, are believed to be 'vexatious' when they are not. I think that sometimes professionals muddle the term 'vexatious' with 'aggressive' or 'vicious'. Within transactional analysis, the Drama Triangle (Karpman 1968) highlights the dynamics between organisations and individuals seeking a service:

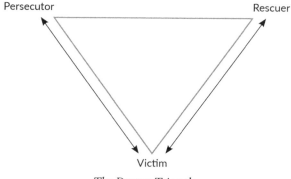

The Drama Triangle

A parent seeking support with the management of their child might approach children's services believing they will be provided the support they need to manage their child. They are effectively looking to a parent body to intervene and help. Sometimes a social care assessment is forthcoming, and often parents are told their child does not meet the eligibility criteria for assessment, or there is a move into the realms of parental blame. When this happens, statutory agencies can inadvertently adopt the role of Persecutor, with the parent(s) feeling they are the Victim. Consequently, parents might decide that they have no option, other than to step into the Persecutor position by making a formal complaint against the professional and/or the organisation. As the statutory organisation has a position of power, there can be a determination to divert attention away from meeting the needs of the child, and to malign the actions of the parent. This can create the interplay of Persecutor and Victim roles between the two parties until a resolution is achieved, sometimes with the parent engaging legal representation to adopt the Rescuer position because they have exhausted their capacity to continue without specialist support.

Not letting the child be seen on their own

A high proportion of neurodivergent children experience anxiety which can be so extreme that they are diagnosed by a specialist clinician as having a generalised anxiety disorder. Sometimes a child is so anxious that they cannot speak (selective mutism). The presentation known as

PDA includes a person resisting and avoiding the ordinary demands of life; using 'social' strategies as part of the avoidance; appearing sociable but lacking some understanding; experiencing intense emotions and mood swings; appearing comfortable in role play, pretence and fantasy; focusing intently (often on other people); and a need for control. Even the simplest of requests or expectations, including pleasurable activities and pursuits, can elicit a fight, flight or freeze response in a child because of the intensity of their anxiety (The PDA Society 2022). Very often, autistic parents will be sensitive to their child's anxiety, and yes, there might be instances when they are fearful of how an inexperienced professional might misinterpret what their child has said. I have met children who have completely masked their real feelings and have sought to present what they believe I want to hear in their efforts to end the meeting as quickly as possible.

Talking for the child/child repeatedly referring or deferring to the parent

An anxious parent, who is anxious for their child, might seek to talk 'for' them because of their need to explain what is going on. A common feature of neurodivergent parents can be their need to give all the details, to ensure what they are saying is accurately interpreted by the listener. As an autistic woman, I can relate to this as there have been many occasions when my supervisor has said, 'Cathie, I don't need all the details.' A neurodivergent child might feel very anxious about talking to an unknown professional, and they really might not know what to say or what is expected from them. Anxiety and fear can elicit a 'freeze' reaction where the child loses their ability to speak. Thus, it is not unusual for them to rely on their parents during assessments and other appointments. A child with a generalised anxiety disorder or the PDA profile might significantly struggle to speak, even when they want to contribute. Furthermore, parents have recounted incidents where a professional has criticised them for talking in front of their child about the difficulties they are encountering, when there has been no alternative option. The parent intuitively knows they must provide an accurate account of their experiences otherwise their concerns will be dismissed or minimised. The irony of this is that when a parent is explicit, their behaviour can be interpreted as exaggeration rather than reality.

Repeated or unexplained changes of school (including to home-schooling), of GP or of paediatrician/health team

There are occasions where a parent will endeavour to do all they can to support their child who appears to them to have difficulties managing school, thus seeking practical solutions rather than blatantly seeking to evade authority. When successive schools do not meet parental expectations, one option is to consider home-schooling, which again can be viewed with suspicion by professionals. If a parent believes a medical professional is not taking their concerns seriously, they might exert their right to request a second opinion or pay privately for an independent assessment. However, changing a child's school and seeking good clinical assessments and support does not equate to child abuse.

Factual discrepancies in statements that the parent makes to professionals or others about their child's illness

Many children and young people I have assessed are not fine in school, although this has not been recognised by their teachers. Parents have provided numerous accounts of being criticised and judged by education professionals because they are asserting the possibility that their child is possibly neurodivergent. Consequently, this leads to parent blame as teachers claim 'She's fine in school', with the underlying message being 'The problem is at home'. Recent research highlights how autistic girls are very skilled at masking or camouflaging their differences whereby they present or perform social behaviours to meet the expectations of their neurotypical peers.

However, when they arrive home all their pent-up 'holding it together' comes out, and their distress is apparent. Tony Attwood (1998) refers to this phenomenon as the 'Jekyll and Hyde' character. In relation to parents being accused of making up their child's physical illness, on two occasions I have worked with two autistic parents of children who have survived cancer; both were individually accused of giving professionals misleading information about their child's illness which led to accusations of FII, despite them providing evidence to the contrary.

Parents pressing for irreversible or drastic treatment options where the clinical need for this is in doubt or based solely on parental reporting

One important matter which is becoming increasingly recognised in autistic people is gender dysphoria. This is where a child or young person expresses incongruence between their assigned gender at birth and their experienced gender. However, the co-occurrence of autistic people and gender dysphoria presents challenges with diagnosis and treatment because of the complexities of 'social, adaptive, self-awareness, communication, and executive functioning' (Strang *et al.* 2018b, p.107). Most child and adolescent services across the UK do not offer the clinical specialists who are trained to support young people questioning their gender identity. Sometimes parents have opted to pursue a private assessment with the young person deciding to accept hormone treatment to support the transition to their identified gender. Understandably, professionals often express great concern about this type of life-changing treatment; however, it does not equate to FII. In other situations, I know of parents being accused of FII when they have privately funded lifesaving treatment abroad because it has not been available within the UK. I doubt any qualified, registered doctor anywhere in the world would act upon the instructions of a parent without forming their own clinical judgement based on clear evidence.

Using transactional analysis to explain the dynamics which can occur between parents and children's social care

When a parent contacts children's social care requesting an assessment of their child, it is usually because they are experiencing difficulties meeting their child's needs, or because they want a social care assessment to support their child's EHCP. In Wales, this is known as 'additional learning needs (special educational needs)'. In seeking support, the parent might well have exhausted all other options and be possibly questioning their ability to provide good enough parenting. At this point, they might be coming from an 'I'm not-OK, You're-OK' position in relation to social care.

At the heart of transactional analysis is the ego-state model which describes a person's behaviours, thoughts and feelings at any given time (Stewart and Joines 2012, p.12):

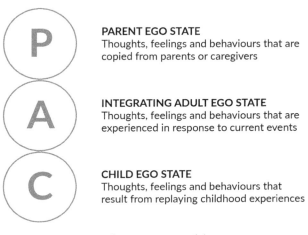

PARENT EGO STATE
Thoughts, feelings and behaviours that are copied from parents or caregivers

INTEGRATING ADULT EGO STATE
Thoughts, feelings and behaviours that are experienced in response to current events

CHILD EGO STATE
Thoughts, feelings and behaviours that result from replaying childhood experiences

The ego-state model

When a parent is in contact with children's social care, they might believe they are communicating from their Adult position, but may subconsciously be in their Child ego state, replaying childhood experiences such as expecting professionals to listen, understand and support them. Children's social care becomes the Parent with the hope that a social worker's role entails supporting their family whilst they are in crisis. When this does not happen, a parent's expectations can be quashed, and they perceive social workers as the Controlling Parent, because they feel criticised, undermined and blamed for their child's difficulties. When this happens, the parent's reaction may be to step onto the aforementioned Drama Triangle where the relational dynamics are unconsciously played out between the two parties.

The skill of the social worker demands that we work from an 'I'm-OK, You're-OK' stance, recognising parents might need our services and that, with the right support, they will rediscover their own internal resources to manage some of what is happening. In cases where there have been expressions of concern about FII, very often a series of mis-judgements are made by professionals which are not evidence based. For example, an NHS paediatrician who has been complained about by the child's parents might make a safeguarding referral stipulating that they believe them to have FII. Social workers have a duty to screen and adhere to their safeguarding guidelines, but equally they must use their professional discretion to question the motivation behind the initial referral. What can rapidly evolve is a subconscious interprofessional collusion where they perceive themselves as 'I'm-OK' and the parent as 'You're not-OK'. If we return to the Drama Triangle, instantaneously the parent will feel they are the Victim and children's social care adopts the Persecutor position. In their efforts to regain their autonomy, a parent might believe their only recourse is to redress the balance by adopting the Persecutor position and complain about the local authority. This type of action further feeds into the concept by professionals that 'vexatious' complaints equate to a parent having something to hide, particularly as this is one of the recognised criteria for FII. This may well reignite the local authority resuming the role of Persecutor because their primary aim is to protect children from the risk of harm. However, the autistic parent who is now probably experiencing fear and anxiety may feel incensed about the injustice that is happening. Consequently, they will either withdraw and disengage from services, or they will retaliate. Whichever approach they adopt will be further attributed to FII, poten-tially creating an ongoing interplay of Persecutor and Victim. The other position on the Drama Triangle is that of Rescuer. When the Victim feels totally disempowered, believing they do not have the resources to change the situation, they will seek support from another person (Rescuer). This could be a solicitor, an independent social worker or an advocate. Whereas the Rescuer comes from a one-up position believing 'I can or want to fix this', they might undermine parental autonomy by taking over. Their involvement can further fuel the allegations of FII until parents feel they have no other choice than to seek legal help. The Rescuer can seek to 'save' the parent by becoming the Persecutor towards the local authority, or being perceived as persecutory, because they are challenging the allegations made by services about the parent. Another position on the Drama Triangle, which is an equally valid one, is that of the *Bystander* (Clarkson 1987). This is when others witness a parent being victimised and either feel they do not have the power to intervene or make a difference, or they choose not to. Their inaction can contribute to what eventually happens.

Whilst recognising the many strengths and qualities autistic parents have, in these situations their internal resources become incredibly depleted, and a third party does need to intervene. The key factor in all of this is the wellbeing of the child at the heart of the enquiry. If their parent is feeling anxious, stressed and depressed and is experiencing a sense of powerlessness and a lack of hope, this will surely affect the child's emotional health.

The antithesis of the Drama Triangle is the Winner's Triangle (Choy 1990):

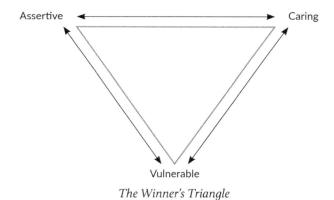

The Winner's Triangle

Assertive supersedes Persecutor whereby parents and professionals articulate their views from an 'I'm-OK, You're-OK' position, with the needs of the child being central to their discussions and neither party seeking to denigrate or discount each other's opinions, even when they disagree. The Rescuer is replaced by the Caring role, whereby the parent's problem-solving abilities are respected, and they are asked what they want and need to help them move forwards. Providing a supportive structure to enable and empower a parent to achieve the right outcomes is far less arduous than acrimony. All too often, when a parent expresses feelings of vulnerability, this can feel as if professionals are using this against them to undermine their parenting capabilities. For example, I have witnessed parents who have been vehemently criticised when they have spoken about feeling anxious and depressed, when the reality is that these feelings are an appropriate response to their situation. Therefore, acceptance of the Vulnerable position can prevent the need to fall into the Victim position. For professionals, this means giving space for parents to express their feelings and encouraging them to ask for the help they feel they need, without judgement, whilst supporting them to implement the steps they need to take to meet their needs. Vulnerable is about the expression of needs, from an Adult ego state, using self-awareness and intuitively addressing issues as they arise. Vulnerability is two-sided, as there might be instances when the social worker needs to honestly express their feelings because this can forge a positive working relationship between the parent and the professional. The importance of the Winner's Triangle is that neither parental nor professional vulnerability is scorned. When mutual trust is achieved, if interpersonal conflicts arise, the positions on the Drama Triangle are made redundant.

If we take the matter further, Hay (1995) has adapted the Winner's Triangle to that of the Potency Pyramid:

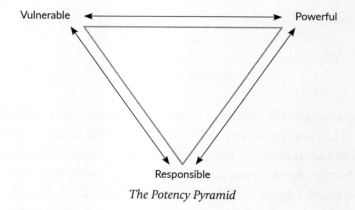

The Potency Pyramid

This supports the concept of individuals showing their vulnerability, whilst maintaining their Adult position, and not discounting that equally they can be Powerful and Responsible to positively influence change. The Potency Pyramid acknowledges the importance of each of us responsibly and simultaneously managing our vulnerability and our power without the need to rescue, persecute or to adopt the Victim role (Hay 2007, pp.92–93).

In situations where children's social care receives a referral specific to FII from an external party, as the lead agency the receiving social worker needs to screen the information provided and ascertain if there is need for input from social care. The designated safeguarding lead must quickly establish whether there is an imminent risk to the welfare of the child and determine whether there is reasonable cause to suspect that a child is suffering, or is likely to suffer, significant harm. Some of the questions needing to be asked include whether a parent or sibling has an existing diagnosis, and is it possible the child has the same condition? Can this be corroborated by another professional/ diagnostician? Has the parent made a complaint against the referring agency or person? Is the parent seeking an EHCP for their child? If a child's parents are separated, are there inter-relational disputes about the child's difficulties?

Once each of these factors has been considered, the social worker needs to decide whether the referral warrants a child protection investigation, or to divert from an immediate reactive investigation with the aim of seeking more information before any further action is taken. Should a home-based assessment be necessary, either under Sections 47 or 17 of the Children Act 1989, when there is any possibility that the child or parent is or could be autistic, it is essential that the professionals undertaking the assessment have appropriate experience and expertise to do this. This should include asking an autistic parent whether any reasonable adjustments need to be made to support them during the interview/assessment process.

A significant percentage of the children and young people I assess are either diagnosed with PDA or present with a demand avoidant profile. There remains interprofessional contentions about whether PDA is a separate diagnosis or an extension of being autistic. The key features of a PDA profile include using elaborate strategies to resist and avoid the everyday demands of life. Sometimes there is a marked demand avoidance, and for other people this is internalised. The underlying issue for demand avoidant children and young people is their intolerance of uncertainty and high anxiety when they feel their autonomy is threatened. For children and young people with PDA or a demand avoidant profile, conventional parenting approaches are not successful. Parents often feel they must tiptoe around their child to prevent the occurrence of behavioural challenges including self-harm, verbal and/or physical abuse, meltdowns and shutdowns.

Implementing the same parental boundaries used with a neurotypical child will increase the child's need to avoid because of their fight or flight reactions due to insurmountable feelings of anxiousness. Whereas most children's social workers are trained to notice and evaluate parental boundaries and attachment difficulties, in these instances a completely different assessment approach is required. Suffice to say, there will be occasions when parental approaches must be questioned, particularly when there is risk of harm to the child. When assessing a child with PDA or a demand avoidant presentation, it is crucial the social worker approaches their assessment with sensitivity and understanding. For example, individuals with PDA are extremely adept at masking their difficulties and will say whatever they believe is expected of them to expedite the assessment process. Their intention will be to get out of the situation as quickly as possible. I applaud the importance of a social worker seeking to ascertain the wishes and feelings of a child, as this is required within the context of assessments and safeguarding. However, in some situations, the views expressed by the child do not necessarily accurately reflect their experiences. I vividly recall being a student social worker in a child protection team and a situation where I sought to do the right thing. I listened intently to the wishes and feelings of a young person who told me how dreadful things were at home and how he needed to get out. My response was to say, 'Don't worry Daniel, we'll get you out of here.' The next time I arrived at his home, I was greeted by a very angry, visibly distressed mother who screamed at me because the child had been 'playing' me to see how I reacted. Daniel had obviously sensed my lack of experience and naivety. Suffice to say, I apologised, and we regained a positive working relationship until my placement ended.

Summary

FII is not a diagnosis and is not to be confused with the rare diagnosis of FDIoA. When a referral is received, which either specifies or infers FII, a cautious evaluation of the evidence supporting this claim is required, in line with the recently published 'Fabricated or Induced Illness and Perplexing Presentations: Abbreviated Practice Guide for Social Work Practitioners (Long *et al.* 2022).

There can be ulterior motives where other professionals can consciously or inadvertently seek to persecute an autistic parent who has dared to question or challenge their authority. This needs to be considered as part of the decision-making process in the context of whether there is a need for a child protection enquiry. When I have asked parents 'What needs to change?', their response is usually that professionals need more training in understanding autistic people and for them to not automatically impose neurotypical expectations when working with autistic parents, or those parents who are possibly neurodivergent. With never-ending cutbacks in local government funding, it is inevitable that there will be an ongoing reduction in the pool of resources social workers can access to support children in need. Rather than professionals 'gaslighting' parents who are requesting a social care provision, the situation demands honesty, where professionals work alongside autistic parents and their children whilst carefully explaining the limitations of what they can offer, and thus seeking to work with the parent to devise and plan strategies which will work.

It is not about sending an autistic parent on another parenting course, but it might be funding some short-term expert support to make the most of the existing strengths within the family. One of the most important aspects of being a proficient social worker is the ability to listen to and connect with parents, where we work with them, whilst not necessarily knowing the outcome. Instead, we walk alongside them, neither rescuing nor persecuting, and coming from a place of 'I'm-OK, You're-OK'. It is about being the professional who cares, the expert practitioner who can listen and evaluate a barrage of conflicting information to arrive at an informed decision, based on fact not opinion, refusing to be the Bystander, and thus standing up for what we believe to be rightful and just.

CHAPTER TEN

The Experience of Autism within the BAME Community

This chapter has been written with the help and support of Venessa Bobb. Venessa is a black woman, an autism awareness advocate and the mother of autistic children. She supports autistic people from the Black African, Black Caribbean, Asian and minority ethnic communities and is the founder of A2nd Voice CIC, an organisation which works with the autistic community, and Autism Thrives Service, which works with professionals.

Venessa has worked with a number of organisations, raising awareness of cultural inequalities and issues that face non-white autistic people, including *SEN Magazine*, BBC Radio 4, the National Autistic Society and Premier Radio (Christian News).

She has faced a variety of challenges over the years, some of which are outlined in this chapter. She attributes her strength to her faith, which is extremely important to her.

This chapter aims to raise awareness of the issues facing black families when they try to seek assessment and support for their children and explores some of the cultural influences that impact upon this process.

Research into the experiences of black autistic children and their families

A brief report, written by Straiton and Sridhar (2022), highlighted the challenges for black autistic individuals and their families in obtaining accurate and timely assessments and high-quality care. They studied the experiences of families in the US and urged clinicians to approach their work with 'cultural humility' (p.2). The authors also noted the need to adopt an ethos that takes into account the impact of the intersectionality of race, disability status and social resources upon quality of life.

The authors go on to discuss that, in the US, anti-black racism has a significant impact upon the assessment and diagnostic process for black autistic people. They report high levels of misdiagnosis of black autistic children and state that these children are 2.6 times more likely to be misdiagnosed compared to white children. Many black children receive a diagnosis of 'adjustment disorder' or 'conduct disorder' according to Mandell *et al.* (2007) despite little actual evidence to suggest that black autistic children are any more likely than white children to display what Mandell *et al.* refer to as externalising behaviour (aggression and/or hyperactivity). Mandell *et al.*'s paper also highlighted that black children often had to wait significantly longer before being assessed, despite displaying a similar level of difficulty to their white counterparts. They concluded that racism in the form of misconceptions and stereotypes were often contributing factors to these delays. Straiton and Sridhar (2022) noted that providers of autism assessment services often attributed this delay to black parents having neither the resources or the motivation to seek earlier assessment for their child.

Lovelace *et al.* (2021) also wrote about the issues of the intersectionality between race, culture and autism stereotypes upon the ability of black women and girls to access both assessment and culturally appropriate therapeutic approaches.

There is an acknowledgement that, in the US, current prevalence estimation methods for autism do not allow for an accurate count of black autistic women and girls. The CDC (Centers for Disease Control and Prevention) initially stated that prevalence rates for autism are measured by both gender and race. However, later research highlighted that this was not happening at a federal level. The Autism Coordinating

Committee's '2019 Summary of Advances in Autism Spectrum Disorder Research' (published in IACC 2020) highlighted 20 articles, not one of which directly addressed the issue of autistic individuals from marginalised groups.

Lovelace *et al.* (2021) further discuss the American statistics with regard to prevalence rates for autism which is cited as 1:54 (Maenner *et al.* 2020). Baio *et al.* (2018) cite almost identical prevalence rates for black children. However, it does not appear that this similarity in prevalence rates is currently (in the US) translating into diagnoses or subsequent access to therapeutic support. In a study carried out in 2014 (Pierce *et al.* 2014) it was reported that in 72 per cent of articles published in three well-known autism journals, no mention of race or ethnicity was made and 54 per cent of the articles published did not consider race and/or ethnicity when discussing their findings.

Despite the barriers that clearly exist in terms of accessing assessment and diagnosis or ensuring culturally appropriate assessment models are used, Ramclam *et al.* (2022) identified a number of cultural and familial strengths within the black community: namely parenting practices that emphasise the importance of mutual respect, independence, protection of and advocacy for children. Faith was also identified as a strong protective factor for many.

Black caregivers of autistic children in the US were reported to rely upon support from their community and within the extended family. This was said to include reporting initial concerns, when going through the process of engaging with professionals and after diagnosis.

Kandeh *et al.* (2020) noted the limited amount of research that is available about how autism is experienced in the black and minority ethnic population within the UK. They noted that many autistic persons globally experience challenges. However, when low levels of autism education and awareness, and cultural and religious beliefs combined with stigma, are factored in, they argue that families can find themselves in 'intolerable, and even dangerous' situations, especially in communities where autism is perceived as a 'punishment from God' (p.166). Autism Voice is a parent-led, not-for-profit organisation established in the United Kingdom in 2013 by a black parent of an autistic child, who was struggling to access support and recognition within their East

London Community. It aimed primarily to deliver culturally sensitive information about autism and has been working ever since to achieve this aim and organised the first Autism Voice UK Symposium in 2018 along with the Participatory Autism Research Collective (PARC) and the Critical Autism and Disabilities Research group based at London South Bank University. The aim of this symposium was to seek the views of the BAME community and ultimately to raise public awareness of the issues faced by autistic people from BAME backgrounds. The symposium also highlighted the need to promote a better understanding of the EHCP process and how to access services (particularly those which may improve opportunities for independence in adulthood).

Martin and Milton (2017) emphasised the role of autistic people as key stakeholders who have huge expertise and knowledge to bring to their communities. Stakeholder involvement in terms of disseminating information was seen as one of the key aspects of the action plan developed by the symposium.

A further important recommendation from the symposium, which, given the other chapters in this book, seems vital, was the suggestion that local authority social services teams across the country need to be made more aware of how the BAME community operates, particularly with regard to care arrangements.

A final point that was noted by participants at the symposium was that there is no word for autism in some of the languages spoken with the BAME community. This was reported to lead to a 'linguistic disconnect' (Kandeh *et al.* 2020, p.7).

The paper by Kandeh *et al.* (2020) also highlighted the results of a study conducted by Slade (2014) on behalf of the National Autistic Society that explained the challenges faced by BAME communities within the UK, specifically those relating to cultural and religious perspectives. Slade explored the various cultural barriers for BAME families both in seeking, and subsequently accepting, a diagnosis of autism for their children. These included a lack of accurate information, religious beliefs and the perceived stereotypical views of schools and local authorities when considering the behaviour of children from BAME backgrounds. The Kandeh *et al.* (2020) study helpfully summarised these key cultural beliefs; they reported that in Nicaraguan and many South American cultures autism and other types of impairment/difference are not even acknowledged. Indeed, an autistic child might be viewed as a 'Gift from God'. In contrast, Kandeh *et al.* noted that in Korean and Ghanaian communities, autistic children are viewed with shame.

Hussein (2021), as part of a doctoral thesis, adopted a phenomenological analysis approach to elicit the experiences of young people who were autistic from a BAME background. Her study highlighted that whilst there were similarities between the experiences of BAME and white autistic individuals in terms of themes identified (such as awareness of self and autism, relationships with peers and the importance of positive relationships), there were also notable differences. Hussein's study highlighted that there were some key experiences that were unique to BAME individuals as a result of their racial and cultural identity.

One of the participants in the study was an autistic Asian woman. She referred to her faith and her belief that 'God had created her this way' with several references to the 'Will of Allah' (Hussein, p.81). She also referred to the fact that, as a child, she had heard herself referred to as a 'retard' (Hussein, p.83) and also stated that she had heard autistic people being referred to, within her community, as 'crazy' (Hussein, p.83).

Another participant, a young Asian man, also noted that 'in traditional India, [autism is] viewed as retardism, it's viewed as you being a failure to your family' (Hussein, p.101). The expectations of family were also discussed at length, particularly the Indian cultural expectation of the roles which Asian children are often expected to conform to (such as doctor, lawyer or businessman), and the young person referred to children being 'berated' within the home environment, if they are unable to achieve a role like this (Hussein, p.106). It was, however, noted that there appeared to be somewhat better understanding in British Asian families, compared to more traditional Indian families.

Another young person mentioned the challenge of not having words to describe autism.

In terms of religious considerations, Slade reported that the two main religions followed within the BAME community where a religious element was apparent were Christianity (mostly followed by the Black African and African-Caribbean community) and Islam (followed by the majority of the South East Asian population).

In the African-Caribbean community, there was reported to be a belief amongst some individuals that autism is caused by demonic spirits and that the way to rid the child of these spirits was through practices such as exorcism.

When these types of belief are combined with commonly held beliefs about autism, alongside cultural stereotypes (such as a gendered acceptance that boys may speak later than girls, and an acceptance that a certain amount of 'boisterous' behaviour is to be expected in boys), it can, and does, lead to families delaying seeking support for their children. Another particularly pertinent cultural belief is that of eye contact. Making direct eye contact with adults in certain communities is seen as rude or disrespectful. Therefore, an unwillingness to make eye contact seen in an autistic child might not be noticed. (Although the importance or relevance of eye contact in autistic persons has been challenged by many, it remains a focus of many autism assessments).

Venessa was kind enough to share her story with me in the hope of highlighting the challenges faced by black autistic families in the United Kingdom.

VENESSA'S STORY

She has three children, one boy and two girls. Her two youngest children are diagnosed as autistic, and her older daughter is still awaiting an official diagnosis. She reported that her son's difficulties were initially more obvious than her daughters'. However, she faced a long battle to secure a diagnosis for him.

The first thing she noticed was his failure to sleep and his unusual eating habits. She then noticed that he would avoid both noise and the sun. Her husband at that time refused to acknowledge that something may be 'wrong' with him.

He started school at a black Christian school that had a reputation of being good with diverse children. School noted that his speech was not clear and that he always played alone. There were also concerns about his behaviour at this time. A speech and language therapist saw him and suggested that he may have ADHD. He was ultimately diagnosed with autism and ADHD.

However, Venessa quickly realised that this diagnosis, within her community, was seen as a 'white disease'. There was a degree of shame in having a child with this type of difficulty, and there was talk of 'supernatural forces', 'getting rid of the devil' or 'praying it out'. There was also a real lack of knowledge about autism; many still believed that it was due to the MMR (Measles, Mumps and Rubella) injections, despite this having been comprehensively dismissed by medical professionals. The emphasis was firmly on 'curing' or 'fixing' the child, and behaviour management programmes were often suggested.

Venessa found herself increasingly isolated and judged. This became more intense when her son began to display increasing levels of challenging behaviour, where he often became physically aggressive towards her and his siblings. When she reached out for help from social care, she quickly found that her parenting was questioned. She was accused of not being able to set appropriate boundaries and was told that her 'mental anxiety' was exacerbating her son's behaviour. At no time did she feel that any practical support was offered to her.

When Venessa's two daughters also began to experience difficulties, these were, once again, attributed to her parenting, or it was assumed that they were simply copying the behaviour of their brother. One daughter was sent to a pupil referral unit on a part-time basis as a last resort, as her primary school did not feel they could support her, and Venessa shared that her daughter was upset by a peer referring to her as 'mentally ill'. Her behaviour was seen as 'childish', 'rude' and 'spoiled' by both professionals who were brought in to support her and members of Venessa's local community. Her other daughter was extremely vulnerable and became pregnant as a teenager. The youngest was eventually diagnosed as autistic and her older daughter was diagnosed as having moderate language difficulties.

Since this time, Venessa has been actively campaigning for black and Asian autistic, dual heritage families. She has produced the list of issues below as being the key areas where understanding and support are needed. Whilst it is important to acknowledge that this list does not have empirical evidence to support it, it does reflect the lived experience of many of the families Venessa has come into contact with, and tried to support, through her advocacy:

1. Misunderstandings and assumptions are frequently made when children display behaviour that challenges. Very rarely is the underlying cause of behaviour explored.

2. Racial prejudice overshadows any diagnosis. Young people are frequently labelled as 'loud', 'feisty' and 'rude'.

3. There is a lack of understanding amongst education and social care staff, and many black autistic children are wrongly labelled as having social, emotional and behavioural problems. There is very little understanding of sensory issues.

4. Black autistic children are frequently given detentions, put into isolation and excluded. Many are sent to pupil referral units.

5. Parents and carers often experience denial from their families and become isolated and alienated. They are often too ashamed to report sibling or parent abuse by the child who is experiencing the challenges. Often there is a breakdown in family relationships and communication, leading to further isolation.

6. Many are scared to report difficulties in case this is used against them to question their parenting.

7. Housing is often overcrowded and there is little space to effectively support sensory needs.

8. There is a poor understanding of the meaning of 'mental capacity', and often vulnerability is overlooked.

9. There are particular issues in this respect in terms of sexual knowledge, vulnerability and teen pregnancy.

Venessa subsequently put together suggestions for how black and Asian dual heritage families might be better supported.

First, she advocates for more specialist training for professionals working within ethnic communities. She also suggests that professional groups need to acknowledge the wide range of traditions, languages and customs that are present within ethnically diverse communities. This might involve connecting with local voluntary and self-help groups to facilitate the process of reaching out to families in a culturally appropriate way.

Venessa also highlights the importance of engaging with the leaders of faith communities as they often provide support and comfort to families. However, it would also be helpful to work with the leaders from different faiths to challenge some of the more negative stereotypes and myths about autism.

CHAPTER ELEVEN

Current Initiatives in the UK to Support Autistic Children and Young People

This final chapter will examine the current initiatives taking place within the United Kingdom to ensure that much needed, more effective and joined-up services are provided for children and young people with 'perplexing presentations' who may otherwise slip through the net and fail to secure an appropriate assessment, diagnosis and support for their challenges. This chapter will also include case studies and personal experiences of individuals and their families who have gone through this process. Although the chapter will report on UK initiatives, they also have relevance in an international context.

In the United Kingdom, it has become apparent that there is an urgent need to review mental health provision for children and young people. This has come into sharp focus following the COVID-19 pandemic and subsequent 'lockdowns' where children and young people were at home for prolonged periods of time, away from friends and face-to-face social activity.

The National Health Service (NHS) carried out a survey that highlighted how the mental health of children and young people had been affected since the previous survey they carried out in 2017 and it appears that there has been a significant increase in the number of young people seeking support for their mental health. This led to the development of the NHS Long Term Plan, which aims to improve services over the coming years.[1]

At the same time, there has been a growing awareness of the number of young autistic people, or those with a learning disability, who are deemed to be 'too complex' for services to support appropriately, many of whom are detained in mental health inpatient units across the country. These units are often many miles away from their homes and families. The actual treatment they receive in such units can be variable. Autism is not, in itself, a mental illness. However, as has been outlined in the preceding chapters, all too often mental health difficulties emerge as a result of young people being misunderstood, misdiagnosed or undiagnosed.

The National Autistic Society in the United Kingdom have campaigned for better services for autistic people across the country. Their aim was, wherever possible, to help people avoid admission to mental health units. Very often distressed or anxious behaviour can be misinterpreted as a sign of mental illness. The Mental Health Act Code of Practice (DHSC MHA 1983, updated 2015 and 2017) states that this should not be the case, or provide grounds for someone being 'sectioned' under the Mental Health Act. In addition, the Code of Practice states that, for autistic people, 'compulsory treatment in a hospital setting is rarely likely to be helpful'.

The NAS guide (NAS 2022) goes on to state that it is vital that all health professionals understand autism (most importantly, people's sensory and communication needs), and services should endeavour to provide a personalised service and avoid a 'one size fits all approach'.[2]

This raises some interesting issues. First, when individuals, autistic or not, are presenting with extremely distressed behaviour (whether this involves aggression towards self or others or self-harm/suicide attempts), the first step is often to intervene using a medical model and psychotropic medication, which is used to support and 'stabilise' the

---

1   www.longtermplan.nhs.uk/online-version
2   www.autism.org.uk/advice-and-guidance/topics/inpatient-mental-health-hospitals/
    autistic-people-and-inpatient-mental-health-hospit/all-audiences

patient. To all intents and purposes, this often involves administering powerful drugs which effectively sedate the individual, thus removing the risk of aggressive or self-harming behaviour. The tragic story of Oliver McGowan, reported in Chapter Six, highlights how this can be a risk for autistic people, who may react in atypical ways to some of the medication used.

Obviously, in theory, once a person is 'stabilised', a treatment plan should then be put in place which should include therapy and a clear formulation of that person's difficulties. In reality, this is often not the case. I have worked in, and visited, a number of mental health establishments and am aware that the actual level of therapeutic support (other than medication) is very variable. This is not a 'name and shame' exercise aimed at any specific provider or hospital, merely an inside view of the challenge faced by providers in providing high-quality, holistic care for autistic patients.

There are several reasons for these challenges in the United Kingdom. First, a number of establishments I have either worked in, or visited as part of my job, have a lack of qualified psychologists and often work with a succession of locum psychiatrists on short-term contracts. In terms of psychological support, it is not clear whether this is a conscious choice to employ fewer, or whether there are country-wide challenges in recruiting psychologists to take on this type of work. Working in such settings can be distressing and emotionally draining, and many professionals become burned out and move onto different types of work.

I recall a time when I was the only qualified psychologist on a site that had more than 25 highly distressed patients, some of whom were autistic. With the best will in the world, completing risk assessments and care plans, attending CPA meetings, assessing and formulating individual difficulties and providing therapy to all of these young people in a standard working week was clearly impossible. In addition, every bed in the hospital was urgently needed, which meant that every room space was precious and needed as a bedroom. This meant that there was no dedicated room for therapy, which resulted in therapy sessions being carried out in corridors or in the communal dining room. Added to this, many of the young people were asleep during the day, due to either the effects of their medication or alterations in their sleep patterns, which made it challenging to see all of them during a working day. This inevitably, perhaps, led to an increased number of 'incidents' of distressed behaviour taking place at night when there were often fewer staff members available to support the young people.

Autistic young people were often placed on general PICU wards along with non-autistic, very troubled young people, so there was no way of assessing their communication needs or sensory issues or making adjustments for these. This often led to them displaying even higher levels of distressed behaviour, due to sensory overload or poor understanding of their communication needs. Many ended up in restraint or even seclusion/isolation as a result.

The second issue adding to the challenges faced in providing appropriate care for autistic young people in mental health units is the issue of recruiting and retaining nurses and support workers/health care assistants. Both often find they are paid more and receive more favourable and flexible working conditions if they work through an agency. For an autistic young person, this can be problematic. Whilst they will often form good therapeutic relationships with regular members of staff who get to know them well, difficulties can emerge once these familiar staff are replaced on a later shift by agency staff who are unfamiliar and may not be aware of their individual needs.

A further issue that faces mental health inpatient units (and to be fair, many community mental health teams) is the issue of training. It has been highlighted earlier in this book that historically psychiatrists received little, if any, training in autism or neurodiversity. Those who specialise in the area may receive some, if they work in learning disability services, but many general CAMHS or adult psychiatrists may not. Fortunately, the Royal College of Psychiatrists have begun to address this issue. A report issued in 2020 (CR228; Royal College of Psychiatrists 2020) was produced as part of a wider drive to improve outcomes for autistic adults. It includes a suggested list of training objectives for psychiatrists and states that all psychiatrists should be able to identify the main features of autism, regardless of the person's age, gender or level of cognitive functioning. This applies to both autism as a single diagnosis, or when it occurs alongside other psychiatric or neurodevelopmental conditions. This is undoubtedly a very positive step, and it is to be hoped that both clinical and forensic psychology training courses also adopt this approach.

There have also been a number of initiatives designed to provide universal training for support staff. Following the tragic death of Oliver McGowan, his mother Paula has campaigned tirelessly for better training in autism for all staff working with young people. In May 2022, the Oliver McGowan Mandatory Training on Learning Disability and Autism passed into law as part of the Health and Social Care Act 2022. Initial pilot programmes have already been run successfully across the United Kingdom, all of which have been co-produced and co-facilitated by autistic people.

This is an incredibly positive step as, in my previous experience of working in this area, it was often difficult to ensure that all staff were appropriately trained. By making it a mandatory requirement for all staff this should be less of an issue and will certainly raise awareness. However, it is still likely that, as in the proposed training for psychiatrists, there will be a need for some members of staff to receive specialist training around more 'complex' presentations. It is to be hoped that this mandatory training is ultimately extended to include other professional bodies (such as court staff and the police).

There are also initiatives in place to raise the profile of support staff and health care workers, who are often the staff with the most day-to-day contact with autistic individuals in hospital. It is hoped that some kind of accredited training programme will be developed going forward.

Unfortunately, many of these initiatives were started prior to the COVID-19 pandemic, which, unsurprisingly, has had a major impact upon both staffing and training within inpatient settings, but as services begin to return to 'normal', these initiatives are being picked up again, though progress is slow.

Another issue which has caused what might have been a short-term, time-limited inpatient stay for some autistic people, particularly adults, has been the lack of coordinated mental health care within the community. Those who do not have a learning disability, as was the case for Emma, whose story is reported later in this chapter, often struggle to find the right community support. At the time of writing this chapter, Emma remains in hospital. For some young people, sadly, there will be no happy outcome or community support. A number of the young people who I have worked with in the community have, very sadly, taken their own lives whilst in inpatient care.

The National Autistic Society reported in 2022 (NAS 2022) that, despite some progress in moving autistic people and people with a learning disability out of hospital settings, the number of autistic people in inpatient facilities had increased. In 2015, it was reported that 58 per cent of those in inpatient units were autistic. Clearly changes in policy and practice are well overdue.

So, how can effective change be achieved and what might assessment and support look like for those individuals who are deemed 'too complex' or 'perplexing' to work with?

Embracing Complexity is a coalition of 38 leading neurodevelopmental and mental health charities working together to think holistically about the estimated 10 per cent of the United Kingdom population who have neurodevelopmental conditions of some kind. Their report published in 2022 (Embracing Complexity 2022) calls for a more joined-up approach to assessment, diagnosis, support and research. They point out that many services are commissioned to only look at one condition (for example, assessment teams for autism are often separate from those who assess for ADHD, even though there is a very high level of comorbidity between the two conditions).

One of the authors, Jan Leavesley, who is the mother of autistic daughters, talks about 'diagnostic overshadowing' where, for example, one of her daughter's ARFID (Avoidant Restrictive Food Intake Disorder), which is a diagnostic condition in its own right, was described by one clinician as simply 'fussy eating'.

She reported that managing referrals and appointments between different services became extremely anxiety provoking (she is also autistic) and exacerbated her fears of being 'fobbed off' by professionals. This is very reminiscent of the experiences of parents discussed earlier in this book, who found that this anxiety ultimately led to accusations of being 'over-concerned' parents or even of fabricating their child's difficulties. The author of the report also discussed how having a team who could holistically assess her child for a number of conditions simultaneously would have been helpful.

The report goes on to discuss ways in which this idea is being piloted across the United Kingdom. Three emerging services were considered, and the challenges they faced – along with successes achieved – were examined. All of these services were specifically set up to assess and diagnose multiple conditions.

Diagnosis and the potential for multi-neurodevelopmental pathways

Accurate and timely diagnosis was identified as the first step towards supporting neurodiverse individuals. The report (Embracing Complexity 2022) was based upon the experiences of 500 people, 60 per cent of whom reported delays in getting assessments or having been 'lost' in the system at some point during their diagnostic journey.

The services who have piloted a more joined-up approach have attempted to establish multi-disciplinary teams who have the ability and capacity to diagnose multiple neurodevelopmental conditions.

Constructing such a pathway was complex and needed to incorporate different age ranges, different levels of professional knowledge and the choice of diagnostic tools and thresholds for referral. However, the rationale behind these pilot schemes was that they could prove to be a valuable route to more timely diagnosis, provide more efficient use of National Health Service resources and improve outcomes for families.

One team, in the East Midlands, set up a service that can assess for both autism and ADHD. In addition, they are able to provide mental health assessments for children and young people who receive a diagnosis from them (this is a huge step forward from the way that many services have historically been set up, where young people have had to wait many months for an onward referral, often having their referral rejected as it was assumed that any anxiety or mental health challenges they experienced were simply 'due to their autism'). Their team consists of psychiatrists, paediatricians, clinical psychologists, nurses and support workers, with additional input from speech and language and occupational therapists.

The team did experience a number of challenges. First, they needed to initially close their waiting list to new referrals whilst the redesign of their pathway took place. This, unsurprisingly, caused some anxiety amongst both professionals and families, and, although waiting times for assessment have now decreased, the services have experienced some issues in terms of staffing.

In terms of success, most young people in this area are now seen for an initial appointment within 7 to 12 weeks, rather than a year, as was previously the case. The team are now also able to offer a range of useful post-diagnostic interventions.

A similar service established in the London area was also evaluated as part of this report. Their pathway involved a single, holistic initial assessment which could highlight a variety of neurodevelopmental conditions. One of the benefits they identified was that families found having their child's difficulties explained to them in a dimensional fashion was helpful in obtaining support for their child, even if diagnostic criteria were not met.

The final service to be evaluated in the Embracing Complexity report was a service in Wales. Like the other services, the initial motivation for setting up a more integrated and streamlined assessment service was an increasing backlog of children and young people waiting for assessment. This service, too, faced challenges in terms of evaluation, due to a lack of funding and the sheer number of children and young people needing an assessment.

The authors of the report noted that as there is a lack of research in the efficacy of any service model, they are not able to recommend, or lobby for, any of the service examples outlined above to be replicated across the whole country. Rather, they aimed to raise awareness amongst professionals, researchers and policy makers as it is clear that the current system, and long wait times, are not meeting needs.

The pathways evaluated were only designed for children. However, the report did highlight that there is a need to address the issue of assessment and diagnosis across the lifespan. They also argue for greater shared responsibility across health, education and social care.

Children and Young People's Quality Improvement Task Force

As mentioned earlier in this chapter, the National Health Service Long Term Plan set out an ambitious target of improving mental health services generally and, more specifically, services for autistic children and young people and those with learning difficulties.

In autumn 2019, the National Quality Improvement Task Force was set up to oversee improvements to specialist inpatient services for children and young people with mental health challenges, autism and learning difficulties. It was originally scheduled for completion in March 2022 but was understandably disrupted by the COVID-19 pandemic. The Oversight Board finished its work in March 2023.

The Task Force also had an Independent Oversight Board, chaired by the previous Children's Commissioner, Anne Longfield, who was given the role of overseeing the improvements in inpatient services. I was fortunate to be invited to be part of this group and have spent my time raising awareness of the particular issues of autistic young people who present with 'complex' or 'perplexing' presentations – fundamentally the group of young people who inspired and have been the subject of this book. Progress has been slow (as many services were adversely affected by COVID, staff shortages/illness were a major challenge), but it has been steady, and there certainly now appears to be a better awareness of the challenges of this group of young people.

In addition, a colleague of mine, Dr Gloria Dura-Vila (a consultant child and adolescent psychiatrist in the NHS), and I co-chair a special interest group (SIG) for professionals (clinicians, education specialists and those working in social care) who are interested in the needs of autistic young people with complex needs. This group is in its early stages, but the aim is to share ideas and good practice and offer peer support and advice.

Finally, there are (again at the time of writing) significant discussions taking place to facilitate further research into this diverse and often poorly understood group of people.

It is to be hoped that stories like Bethany's below will not be the norm in the future.

BETHANY'S STORY

Bethany's case was the subject of a serious incident investigation report (Secretary of State Case Review 2019).

Bethany is a young person who has a diagnosis of autism with the PDA profile, whose case came into the public domain following a concerted campaign by her father Jeremy, who worked tirelessly to raise awareness of her situation. At the time her case was made public, Bethany was being held in a seclusion suite in an inpatient CAMHS service and was being fed her meals through a hatch in the door. This hatch was also her only means of contact with her family, as she was deemed 'too dangerous' to support in any other way.

Bethany's case is an excellent (and painful) example of how a lack of the right type of support for young people presenting with complex needs can lead to outcomes which, at many levels, appear inhumane in a modern civilised society.

Bethany's story began long before she came to the public's attention, and sadly her story is by no means unique. Many other individuals have experienced similar failures in their care.

She first began to display what was seen as 'challenging' behaviour when she was at nursery school. This was followed by multiple school exclusions, requests for support from CAMHS and social care, failed residential placements and, ultimately, involvement with the police and criminal justice system before she was finally sectioned under the Mental Health Act.

Her parents were, like many other parents in similar situations, told that her difficulties were due to 'poor parenting', that they needed to be firmer with her and impose more boundaries.

However, Bethany's parents were not poor parents. They were experienced parents who had raised other children without the same level of challenge. At this point though, they were prepared to try anything and attended all the parenting courses they were offered.

Eventually, and again like many other parents, they were given a diagnosis of 'atypical' autism and it was suggested that a school for children with behavioural, emotional and social difficulties (BESD) would be the most appropriate placement for her. This proved unhelpful as Bethany soon became even more 'disruptive', and ultimately the school decided that they were unable to meet her needs. This resulted in her first contact with the police, who were called to help manage her increasingly aggressive outbursts.

The increase in aggression and violence makes sense in the context of her autism diagnosis, as it always created a predictable response and removed her from a situation that she found intolerable. However, it became increasingly difficult for her family to manage, and they were forced to admit that she was 'beyond their control'. Triggers for her 'meltdowns' were often difficult to predict, and after she jumped out of a window at the family home and assaulted someone who was walking by, she was taken to an assessment and treatment unit (ATU), initially as an informal patient. This was supported by her family, as they felt that it would result in support for both them and her. She was subsequently sectioned under the Mental Health Act and remained there until she was moved to a residential school.

Bethany's father reported that she initially did quite well at this placement, and it was here that they became aware of the PDA profile. When they read the information on the National Autistic Society website about it, the description and the suggested techniques for supporting young people made perfect sense to her parents. However, for the reasons described in previous chapters, because this profile remains under-researched and poorly understood it was not fully accepted by the professionals working with her at this placement, even though it had been demonstrated by her family that when she was at home at the weekend on home leave, 'low demand' strategies, including giving her choice and using humour to deflect 'meltdowns', had proved effective.

At her residential school, Bethany continued to display 'challenging behaviour' and the placement ultimately failed. Bethany's father reports that a further 17 placements followed over the coming years. During this time, Bethany had multiple encounters with the police and was cautioned and charged with assault. When these charges were brought up in court, they were ultimately dropped when her autism diagnosis was explained.

After the failure of these placements, Bethany was once again admitted to an ATU for a medication review and for 'treatment'. Following this second assessment, it was once again felt that her needs would be better met in a bespoke community placement, despite her local authority considering that she may need to be moved to a medium secure unit. For context, there are only a few of these units across the country, and they support the most challenging young people. Further assessment once again deemed that this was unnecessary, and plans were at last put in place to develop a bespoke package of care in her local area. It was also agreed at this point that she was in fact 'complex' and that she did display traits of PDA.

Much time and effort was put into preparing Bethany for this move. Unfortunately, though, the time that this took, and the lack of information that was readily available to Bethany about how and when this would happen and what exactly her new placement would look like, led to a huge increase in her anxiety levels and a consequent re-escalation of her 'challenging' behaviour. She was spending up to 23 hours per day being nursed in seclusion (which was effectively a small cell, with a hatch in the doorway through which her food was passed). This deterioration led the potential provider to withdraw their offer of a placement. This must have been devastating for both Bethany and her family as they had now been travelling many miles every week for years to visit her at various placements.

Reaching desperation point with the apparent lack of progress in securing a more appropriate placement for Bethany, her father began opening up about her issues on social and other media. However, he then found himself faced with a court injunction for discussing Bethany, which then led to a summons to the High Court of Justice in London. Fortunately for the family, the pro bono services of two barristers were secured as a result of the social media interest in her case.

Bethany's father was able to put together a case, which demonstrated long-standing historical issues with regard to her care, sharing multiple reports and documents from reviews. He was also able to demonstrate that Bethany had capacity and was able to consent to her case being shared publicly. This led to the judge recommending that the local authority withdrew their application for the continuation of the injunction, which they did, and it was lifted.

Since this time Bethany has been moved to a community placement that finally meets her needs, and a serious case review (2019) has been carried out which made the following recommendations:

1. All agencies will have a statutory duty to work across health, social care and education to produce an individualised and personalised plan.

2. Individualised crisis response plans will need to be co-produced by parents and young people. There is a requirement for children and young people who have the potential to experience crisis to be on a regional support register.

3. National guidance is to be produced to make sure that seclusion or segregation is only ever used as a last resort. All cases will be subject to review.

4. A review of the health, education and social care workforce will be carried out on a national basis with the aim of identifying the core competencies that are required to support young autistic people.

5. An assessment of the individual's human rights will become a mandatory requirement for both providers and commissioners whenever a young person experiences restricted interventions. This includes when the young person's discharge is unduly delayed.

6. Strategic planning at a national level will allow for the development of bespoke community placements to support young autistic people.

7. Following reports that parents have often been excluded from participating in decisions about the care and support of their children, going forward there will be a focus upon parents as partners.

8. There is strong evidence that hospital environments do not always provide the necessary adaptations for autistic people and do not meet their needs. No young autistic person should be admitted to a mental health establishment without clear evidence of a mental health need and an indication that therapy with clear outcomes will be provided.

9. Further development of the navigator (keyworker) process to act as a coordinator in cases of significant concern.

10. A commitment to ensuring the voice of the young person is heard, including strengthening the role of advocates.

The need for early support and intervention

Perhaps the takeaway message from this book is as simple as the title of this final section. As explained in earlier chapters, there is often both a lack of early support available for families and, in many cases, a lack of understanding about autism. The cornerstone of many clinical psychology and social work training courses is attachment and the protective benefit of ensuring secure attachment to a caregiver. This is undoubtedly true, and there are many examples of how an insecure attachment can lead to later mental health (and behaviour) challenges. Many parenting courses are based upon the principles of programmes such as the Solihull Approach, which emphasises emotional containment, parental reciprocity and behaviour management. However, in the course of my clinical career, I have come across so many families who are effectively broken by the challenges of trying to support a child with complex needs. These are not families who are unable to connect emotionally with their child, or who are unable to implement any kind of boundaries; they are often loving, caring families who are regularly hit, bitten, kicked and scratched by young people in complete distress. Young people who can have 'meltdowns' that last for hours, with no apparent trigger. Families who are unable to enjoy days out of the family home, visit relatives or have any kind of respite. Parents who have to give up work in order to care for a child who is simply unable to attend school, or those who are fighting for the right kind of support in school. These families often have other children whose needs cannot be met because of the challenges of trying to support one child, some of whom are forced into the impossible position of having to separate siblings in order to protect them.

Throughout this book, I have told the, often harrowing, stories of children and young people who have been locked away, misunderstood and misdiagnosed, but it is equally important to acknowledge the needs of their parents. Very often the outside world does not see the challenges that go on behind closed doors at home. Frequently teachers just see the child who turns up for school in pyjamas and with unbrushed hair and make a judgement about that child's parents. What they have not seen is the hour-long struggle that they have had to get to that point. They won't have seen the other children in the family, sitting in the car crying because they are going to be late for school and are worried about getting into trouble. They won't have seen the parents sitting through the long night, trying to persuade a distressed child to go to sleep, then two hours later, get up, washed and ready for school. The stories below, bravely provided by Emma and her mother, Kathryn, show both sides of the story, and for me highlight the urgent need for early support for families, given without judgement and blame. Very often when I meet families for the first time as part of the assessment process for their child, the first hour is spent just listening and hearing their story. For many it is the first time they have been able to be honest about their challenges and admit how difficult it can be. All, without exception, love their children dearly.

EMMA'S STORY

As a neurodivergent person struggling with severe mental health issues I have had the input of countless professionals with varying experience through training and/or understanding. The difference between training and understanding is a vital part of the care which that specific individual can provide but is so rarely taken into account. It is my opinion that these generally go hand in hand, but that the ability to understand is far more important.

Throughout my life I have met many people who are technically trained in autism, at least to that care provider's expectation, but do not understand. Understanding is to an extent intuitive; some people just don't have the ability to understand, but the most important thing to understanding is being open to the concept that you may not understand. Autism is different for each and every individual. There are infinite profiles, and each is entirely unique.

This is unfortunately proven by the failures in support systems. Almost every institution is divided into categories and can only function within those walls, but people don't. To put any individual with mental health issues into a category and essentially prescribe a treatment plan is absurd, but to put autistic people into a category and expect the same support to work with even two individuals just does not work. I was nine when my parents took me to the doctor to ask for help. I remember one freeze frame moment that day. Things at home were getting more and more difficult, and my meltdowns were becoming extreme. Instead of driving me to school they took me to the doctors, and all I remember is when my dad parked the car and I realised they weren't taking me to school. I just remember looking through the window and the fear, the confusion, the anger. I had felt different and just wrong for a long time before, but this was proof that there was something wrong with me. I want to make clear that I don't see having autism as having something wrong with me, but as that terrified little girl that's exactly how it felt. I was scared of myself.

After a course of counselling I was referred to have an assessment, and when I was 11 I was given my diagnosis of autism spectrum disorder. At this time, my parents were advised not to tell me, so I just carried on growing up not feeling normal, being wrong and bad, having to hide everything I felt. My school didn't know about my autism, so I didn't receive any support, but even when I found out about my diagnosis at 14, I didn't want the school to know. I felt that if my teachers found out they would judge me, and it would affect my reputation; I would no longer be this perfect student with good grades and friends. There was no part of me that thought maybe it wasn't purely a bad thing, maybe it was more than something to be embarrassed about and hide away. Autism is just a word. It meant nothing to me, just something different, something wrong with me. I took my first overdose at 15 and was admitted to my first psychiatric unit about a week after. I was there for six months, and my autism was known about, but there was no understanding. I was depressed, that was the problem, not the meltdowns that went on for hours and the shouting that hurt my head so much I hid in the wardrobe. Each time I was struggling they turned the light on, spoke loudly to me when I wouldn't respond and went straight for restraint rather than trying to talk to me and deescalate the situation. They injected me a lot and I now have a complex-PTSD diagnosis because of the trauma.

A hospital environment is challenging under any circumstance, and even more so with autism. As well as the restraints and the injections I was put on a lot of medication that heavily sedated me. Strong antipsychotics and antidepressants, lots of sleep medication and more. When I was discharged and under CAMHS I wasn't in the neurodevelopmental pathway that I should have been. I'm not stereotypically autistic; I can look people in the eyes and am generally articulate. I didn't make the cut. I had multiple courses of therapy that only seemed to make me worse, I was being told time and time again I was just being difficult, I was aggressive and mean, just a grumpy teenager.

The head of the CAMHS pathway I was under was particularly cruel. She refused to accept my ASD diagnosis and eventually stopped allowing me access to therapy. She gave me a psychiatric assessment once to see if I needed to be readmitted into hospital. She told me to grow up, take responsibility for my actions, stop overreacting and acting out of anger. I will never forget that phrase 'take responsibility for your actions'. I have so many flashbacks about that conversation, and it brings me to tears nearly every time I think about it. She denied she said it, she told me my mental health wasn't that bad. Apparently, I had fabricated the conversation. The lady from the crisis team who was also there knew I wasn't lying, but who are people supposed to believe? The mental health team wrote the documents, described my profile. The lack of input from patients into their own care is something I find difficult to understand, but when that care is purely directed by individuals without understanding of neurodevelopmental issues, the chance of appropriate care is slim. My atypical presentation of autism has led to many difficult paths and many difficult encounters with people who aren't properly trained. My care coordinator had no experience in autism and pushed me into difficult situations relating to therapy.

DBT is a form of therapy specifically suited to people with person-ality disorders and specifically not autistic people. I initially had CBT, but I was only allowed 12 sessions. The push for me to do DBT, which I had done with the crisis team and in hospital, was incredibly difficult for me considering my demand avoidant profile, so I discharged myself from the services. This meant I refused to see everyone including the psychiatrist, so one day I simply refused to take my medication. I don't remember that summer at all; apparently I didn't speak for over a month or leave my room. My parents were constantly blamed for my deteriorating mental health, and social services became involved. The chairperson of the child protection meeting saw me beforehand. She drew three lines on the whiteboard. One was me being a teenager, one was me with mental health issues, one was me with autism. She asked me how I knew I was struggling with my mental health issues or not managing my autism. Maybe, she said, I was just being an attention-seeking child who needed more discipline. We were only referred to social services because of the number of times I had gone to hospital after serious self-harm or suicide attempts. There was no help given, only problems and faults being noticed and scrutinised. That meeting broke my mum. I was under the crisis team for a while, but they had no experience in autism and the constant flux of people visiting me was overwhelming.

Communication difficulties are a key part of autism but not always in obvious ways; I can have a conversation with almost anyone and they wouldn't notice any difficulties. Communication is, however, difficult for me, a combination of trusting someone, and being able to say things in a way that can be understood by others, trying to stop people from assuming certain things and knowing what to say when they do. Objectively I can speak clearly in ways that are easily understood, but subjectivity is completely different. To speak about myself and my challenges, this is what I struggle with. A key part of my communication issues is internal. In a way I find it difficult to communicate with myself, knowing what I struggle with and recognising triggers. To try and find the right words to explain to someone something I don't understand is almost impossible. When I talk about myself to others, I have to translate the words in my head to words that make sense to them. Equally the people supporting me must have the ability to attempt to understand what I mean because in times of distress I don't have the capacity to process the high levels of cognition needed to complete the appropriate function of translation. I once had a therapy session where the psychotherapist asked how I felt. This was one of the few occasions I answered without thinking. I felt like a concave, fluffy, yellow circle, much like the shape of a red blood cell. I feel in a different language to others and often in a language I myself don't understand. For someone to plainly ask how I feel is incredibly frustrating because I rarely have any idea. I need help to find the answer, for someone to understand that I may not know, and not think I'm being obstructive. I don't know how many people in CAMHS said that. I just made up the answer. On a scale of one to ten I chose a number underneath five that I found particularly favourable that day. Never four, it's too even and the square of two. I would rather have avoided two as well, but that would have left me with only one and three, which they would have picked up on, only rotating between two numbers.

After my discharge I tried going back to school, but I just couldn't cope. They assigned me a specialist teacher who was the first person I'd ever met who knew anything about autism. She introduced me to the demand avoidant profile of autism and has changed my life. She taught me about meltdowns and shutdowns. She didn't work with an autistic person, she worked with me, helped me. My family and I learnt more about autism and the impacts it can have. We began to realise the importance of understanding and working with my ASD rather than against it. Together we ran some sessions for parents of autistic children, specifically with demand avoidant profiles.

My parents have always been strong advocates for me, and after pushing for me to be put on the neurodevelopmental pathway, with the advice from my specialist teacher I agreed and was able to see a specialist trained psychiatrist, and I was lucky enough for him to offer me therapy. This therapy had no model or structure, which understandably sounds odd, but the therapy was built around me. Each session was completely different based on what my week had been like, and for the first time in years I had the motivation to further look into ideas and concepts he raised in our sessions. He diagnosed me with ADHD and complex-PTSD, recognising within only a couple of sessions what no professional had considered before. This shows the importance of having trained and understanding people to support you because again, much like it had been my experience of discovering my ASD diagnosis, I only understood the stereotype that is projected not only onto society but the individuals within a service who don't have the training and skill to identify different profiles of neurodivergence.

I then enrolled in college to do my A levels, but I was particularly struggling with my mental health, and, after a serious incident, I was excluded within four weeks. My mental health continued to deteriorate, and by summer I was readmitted into hospital; again, there was no consideration of autism or the difficulties of the environment. In September I tried again to go to college, this time with an EHCP which I had mostly written myself with the help of my specialist teacher. My EHCP doesn't have what I suppose are usual recommendations because of my complex profile.

I don't need academic support; I struggle with motivation and the environment. People telling me to do my work has an adverse effect because of the demand avoidance, and I don't want to have special needs. I didn't access student support because I don't want to have problems. I wasn't involved in the decisions, which I found particularly difficult, and after six weeks I had a major incident there and wasn't allowed back. I was sectioned into my third CAMHS unit shortly after. This unit had different issues as I was nearly 18 and would have to transition into adult services.

The planning for transition into adult mental health services is meant to start six months before you turn 18; this transition period is specifically important for people on the spectrum because of the difficulties in change and form of care offered. In that unit the psychiatrist didn't allow me to access therapy. I don't know why, but I wasn't allowed to have therapy. Any mention of autism or support relating to that was out of the question. My stay there was extended by three days after my birthday to give them time to do the transition. The decision was to discharge me, even though in the meeting my dad said I wouldn't be safe at home. The consultant psychiatrist's advice was to leave me outside the council and say it was a medical emergency.

In my county adult mental health services don't have a neurodevelopmental pathway, my psychiatrist had no experience, and my care coordinator knew some people who were trained in autism. I knew more about my autism, how things had to be done slightly differently for me and that it didn't matter who knew about it because at this point my life depended on people understanding. There was no one left to help; the wrong help can be worse than no help at all. I was struggling with my PTSD, and all I had were prescriptions and pills. No therapy, no meetings. In and out of hospital at least once a week, running away and being found by the police. Eventually I was admitted to my first adult unit, a female acute unit. They didn't know anything about autism, but they didn't want to either. They would say they couldn't help me until I helped myself, so I would bang my head until I fell over while they just watched.

One of the obstacles I've faced time and time again is my being involved in my care. I am very particular about care plans and what I believe is right and wrong. I'm not afraid to tell someone they are wrong and not in a rude way. If someone listens to me I will listen to them, but if they don't listen then I get carried away because it doesn't matter what I say. It was the period building up to my admission, and in that unit, that the idea of having a personality disorder was speculated. The psychiatric assessments that have to happen to be discharged from general hospital after an admission relating to mental health issues are carried out purely by people with no experience in autism from the crisis team that focus specifically on DBT, a form of therapy that is most effective with personality disorders. From the female acute unit, I was transferred to a unit where I had the fortune of working with Dr Judy Eaton. The assessment that was carried out was full and multidimensional; the nursing staff that worked with me had a better understanding of my needs but were also able to pick up on signs that I was struggling. Not your typical signs of stress but my signs of stress. Again, there was that therapeutic space but not a void to be filled by my initiation, a space to give me the opportunity to have the therapy in the way I needed it. The psychiatrist there confirmed that I did not have a personality disorder.

Sadly though, the hospital closed, and I was discharged with the intent of being readmitted to another, suitable unit, within a matter of weeks. In the months that followed I saw no one from the mental health team. My mum was supporting me alone whilst working a full-time job. I don't know how many times I attempted to take my life or self-harmed to a life-threatening degree, but one example I can give you is that I was found unconscious in the woods after cutting my neck. No Mental Health Act assessment was carried out. For three months I was at home with only my mum to support me. I saw no one from the mental health or social health services. Because of the failures of the system my mum was forced to take the legal route, and I was only admitted to my current placement after it was clear my case would have been taken to the High Court. Coincidences do exist in this world, and I wish this was one of them. The day I was sectioned to my current hospital was the first time I had ever met my care coordinator despite being under his care for over a year. I am 19, this is my sixth mental health hospital and I take over 30 tablets a day. Despite the gradual improvement in understanding my autism and sensory profile, there are still sometimes catastrophic failures in my care. I am lucky to have the ability to have input and involvement in my care. Some people have said that I surely wouldn't want to be just another statistic. This is very true. I am more than one in seven billion, each atom alone in my body is more than one in seven billion and together that's a very large number, but that's not the point. My point is that to the mental health service and throughout my care, that is all I have been: a statistic. Something, or someone, to categorise. The aspects of my care that have helped me have all been person centred and adapted to me; that's what every individual deserves.

KATHRYN'S STORY

One of the most difficult decisions to make when telling someone what we as a family have been through with local health services as a result of my daughter's autism and her connected mental health difficulties is deciding what to leave out. There have been so many failures and so many traumatic incidents that it is too much to take in. After a point, anyone who hasn't experienced it for themselves simply stops believing me. I have come to think that this is because, if you do believe me, your faith in the institutions you would need to rely on should you or your loved ones experience a mental health crisis would be utterly undermined. That is terrifying. What if there is no safety net? It is so much easier to think that this can't be true, or it must be something about us, or that it would be so different if you were doing it.

And where should I begin? This has been going on for so many years now. Should I start at my daughter's diagnosis, aged 11? How different things could have been if we had received support then from people with a background in autism who could help her – and us – to understand her presentation and specific needs. But there was nothing; as my daughter was academically a high achiever she was diagnosed and immediately discharged. What about when I got back in touch with mental health services when she was 14 because I could see she was struggling, and I couldn't seem to help her? Proper support at that time could have been transformative. But a decision was made by our local services – without our knowledge or input and, astonishingly, without any input or assessment by a specialist in autism – that she did not warrant referral to the neurodevelopmental pathway. That fixed the course to my daughter's first life-threatening overdose, aged 15, and five months in a mental health hospital. And it was only after her discharge from there that things started to go really wrong.

I can't start at the end, because we are still living with the failures in the system and lack of support. My daughter is currently in another mental health hospital. This is her sixth one now, and she is only 19. It isn't good there. She isn't receiving any psychological therapy. The hospital psychologist told my daughter she wasn't able to communicate with her after the only session they had. My daughter didn't ever see her again, and anyway the psychologist has now left the hospital. Hospital management (again no experts in autism – there is a definite strand which runs through my daughter's story) have subsequently suggested that she doesn't actually need therapy whilst she is in hospital anyway, and this is something to consider after discharge. Only...how then can her mental health improve to enable her to be discharged? Hospital is not a therapeutic environment in itself if you are autistic. And the many, many drugs she is taking are keeping her stable but not helping her to get better. But when I ask these questions, I am told I am being difficult, and my expectations are too high. The hospital management, our local services – the NHS trust, our local authority, the clinical commissioning group (CCG) – all have me noted as a difficult parent because I keep asking difficult questions. I have actually read this in my daughter's medical notes. Yet...she has been in her current hospital for eight months now, and there is no plan in place for her ongoing care, no plan for treatment, no plan for discharge. The commissioners don't hold the hospital to account, and there is no one to hold the commissioners to account. So, if I stop fighting, what hope can she have for the future?

It might be better to focus on some particular periods in time instead. The transition period from child to adult mental health services could be one. I say 'transition' though really it was just an ending and a transfer. But the most recent of the periods which I have nightmares about is the time before my daughter's admission to her current hospital.

For a period last year, my daughter was in a hospital which did seem to be helping her. It wasn't perfect. Certain things like support with washing clothes and cleaning rooms appear to be a challenge in all mental health hospitals in the UK. But she was having therapy from someone with a real understanding of autism and demand avoidance, which is my daughter's presentation. She had started receiving treatment for her PTSD. The psychiatrist understood autism. My daughter's mental health was getting better. And then the hospital closed. Its funding structure broke down, and it ran out of money. There was less than a week to decide where she should be moved to. I was told by our NHS trust that the options were for her to be admitted to an acute ward or for me to bring her home whilst an alternative specialist placement was commissioned.

My daughter has been in the local acute ward before. It is truly a type of hell. The clinicians have no understanding of autism, and what constitutes care has been stripped down to the bare minimum. On the whole, the staff watch the patients but don't interact with them. And if the sensory overload leads to an autistic meltdown there is an isolation room. When my daughter was there, she spent three days in the isolation room after having a meltdown. After that, a nurse who had clearly had enough let me in to see her. The room's vivid green paint was chipped and flaking. The floor was hard and beige. The window barred and smeared. There was a harsh, blue plastic-covered rectangle for a bed. One pillow and a hospital blanket. Nothing else. Not even a sheet. Two members of staff sat just outside watching my daughter as if they were looking at a particularly boring TV show. Talking to each other but making no attempt to communicate with her. She was curled up on the plastic rectangle moaning quietly. She hadn't eaten, drunk or been to the toilet since she had been put in the room. The only positive thing was that no one attempted to stop me when I said I was taking my daughter home. I still have flashbacks to seeing her in that state, in that place.

There was no way she could go back there. So, I had some long discussions with the clinical director of our NHS trust and the CCG and agreed she could come home so long as community services were in place to provide support alongside me whilst a new specialist hospital was found as a matter of urgency. The hospital psychiatrist and the psychologist she had been working with were commissioned to see her remotely for an hour each week to provide continuity. It actually felt quite good to be bringing her home for a bit. But the weeks began to pass. The online sessions took a while to set up and couldn't be arranged for every week. The promised crisis plan didn't materialise. We were informed a community care coordinator had been appointed, but we didn't know who they were or have their contact details; we certainly didn't hear from them. We were informed a community psychiatrist had been appointed but that they had no expertise in autism and were not going to have any clinical input into my daughter. Again, no contact details and no contact. We seemed to have been cut adrift. My daughter's mental health began to deteriorate. She began to self-harm. She had been under section in a secure hospital with a team of staff to help her day and night and one-to-one support between 5 and 10 p.m. There was now just me in a family home. I started to send increasingly desperate emails to the trust, the local authority and the CCG: '[My daughter] now feels a bit abandoned as it doesn't feel as if there is a plan.' 'The longer things go on without anything else in place the more likely [my daughter] is to get frustrated and the more anxious she becomes. Family members are bringing food etc. but that is also not sustainable for much longer and there is no crisis management plan in place.' 'I am going to need some support to enable me to leave the house a couple of times a week for shopping, collecting meds, etc.' And then, inevitably, 'I am afraid [my daughter] found the pack with her weekly meds yesterday afternoon and took the lot.'

This was a life-threatening overdose, and my daughter was in hospital for four days. A Mental Health Act assessment was arranged. My daughter's medical notes show that it was at this point, finally, that the commissioners contacted some specialist hospitals. What I was told was that no bed was currently available apart from the local acute ward. I sent desperate emails:

> ...her situation at home was allowed to drift without sufficient support being made available for too long and the overdose was the inevitable consequence. There simply must be an alternative now to compounding all the errors that have gone before by sending [my daughter] back to an acute ward to be managed by staff who simply do not have sufficient training in and understanding of her ASD.

And then the Mental Health Act assessment took place. It focused on where my daughter might be sent if she were to be sectioned. It ignored what would happen if she was not. My email at the end of that period sets out what happened:

> [My daughter] has now had the Mental Health Act assessment and has not been sectioned. This was in large part because everyone acknowledged there was no appropriate treatment available. The likelihood was that she would be sent to an acute bed out of area which would probably be no better than the ward where she had been before and this would be damaging. [My daughter] has agreed to engage with the crisis team, but we know that model of support is not good for someone on the autistic spectrum and there is a need to be realistic about her risk at home. I said when she came from hospital that the longer she continued at home, the greater the risks, and the more likely it would be that I would need additional support. I now need that support to be initiated because I am working during the day so unable to monitor her to the extent that it is now apparent she needs. I have been unable to leave the house for shopping or exercise or to deal with medication for six weeks now, and this is impacting on my health. I will also need assistance managing her medication going forward as she now knows where it has been stored, and I don't feel safe having the quantity I need to have access to in the house. We all want [my daughter] to be able to stay at home safely whilst an assessment is carried out and

suitable care is sourced. But I do now need some help if I am to manage this any longer.

My daughter and I returned to the family home. She received a telephone call from the local crisis team. Then – nothing. A week later – still nothing apart from an arrangement with a local pharmacist to have my daughter's medication delivered to me on a weekly basis. Another week – still nothing. And by nothing, I mean really nothing. No contact from local services, no contact from the care coordinator (we never had any contact from the care coordinator), no contact from anyone apart from the psychologist and psychiatrist from the closed hospital who weren't providing therapeutic support for my daughter any more but were still there and also frustrated at the lack of progress or local support. Another week – another overdose, another hospital visit, still nothing. I contacted my daughter's solicitor, and a letter was sent. Then, at last, we were informed there was to be a 'professionals' meeting' (which we have learned basically means a meeting which the family can't attend) and then that a hospital was to be approached to see if a bed could be arranged. An online assessment took place. And then, again...nothing. Another solicitor's letter was sent, longer this time and setting out our proposal for what my daughter and I needed to support us. Finally, the solicitor sent a formal letter setting out that we intended to bring legal proceedings.

As before, this produced a response – we were informed that another professionals' meeting was to be held. Then, magically, we were offered a meeting with even more senior people at the trust and the CCG. They were going to look again for specialist hospitals. There were more discussions, more meetings. But – nothing happened. More support was talked about, but it didn't materialise. Draft plans were emailed around but never finalised. After a further two weeks we issued legal proceedings seeking an expedited hearing. But we were too late; it was half term, and the court wasn't sitting for yet another week. My daughter's mental health had been steadily deteriorating all this time. I was still managing on my own at home, trying to watch her day and night. I was unable to leave the house, unable to sleep, barely able to eat. Finally, that weekend I fell asleep in exhaustion during the afternoon. I woke when my telephone rang. My daughter had been found in some nearby woods by someone walking their dog. She had climbed over the garden gate, gone to the woods and cut her throat with a blade. Fortunately, she was still alive. The person who found her had called an ambulance and then me. The following week a further Mental Health Act assessment was called, and my daughter was sectioned and admitted to the hospital where she is now. She had been home for four months, during which time we had attended hospital eight times due to serious self-harming incidents or suicide attempts. I have a list of these which I prepared for the purposes of the legal proceedings – overdoses, increasingly serious lacerations; one time she locked me in the garden and poured a kettle of boiling water over her arm.

Each time we attended hospital, and after her physical injuries were treated, we saw the hospital psychiatric team. Each time they expressed shock at the situation we were in but said there was little they could do apart from contacting our community team. Apart from one short telephone call, once, we didn't hear anything from our community team after any of these incidents.

Writing this has made me angry again as well as sad. But it has also reminded me why I am so mistrustful of our local services, and why it is right that I should keep on fighting. Because my daughter, and others like her, deserve better.

Epilogue

I am aware that some of the content of this book is hard to read, and for some of the young people discussed, tragically, it is too late to help them. Others continue to suffer from the trauma that they have experienced.

However, it would not be right to end this book on a negative note. There are also some very positive stories to report. One of the contributors is an extremely talented artist and has used her experiences to create some amazing artwork. Others have become advocates for the autistic community and provide training and support. One has written a fabulous book of poetry in which she explores her feelings.

On an institutional and national level, there have been a number of documentaries shown on national television in the United Kingdom during the writing of this book which have begun to expose practices within inpatient units, which were, to put it frankly, abusive in many cases. Many of the young people featured in these documentaries were autistic, and, as a result, changes are being made.

Awareness of the complex ways in which neurodiversity and the environment can interact is growing and it is to be hoped that, in future, life will be better for both these individuals and their families.

References

Al-Attar, Z. (2020) Autism spectrum disorders and terrorism: how different features of autism can contextualise vulnerability and resilience. *The Journal of Forensic Psychiatry and Psychology 31*, 6, 926–949.

Allely, C.S. and Faccini, L. (2019) Clinical profile risk and critical factors and the application of the 'path towards intended violence' model in the case of mass shooter Dylann Roof. *Deviant Behaviour 40*, 6, 672–689.

Allison, C., Auyeung, B. and Baron-Cohen, S. (2012) Towards a brief 'red flags' for autism screening: The Short Autism Spectrum Quotient and the Short Quantitative Checklist in 1,000 cases and 3,000 controls. *Journal of the American Academy of Child and Adolescent Psychiatry 51*, 2, 202–212.

Anthony, L.G., Kenworthy, L., Yerys, B., Jankowski, K. *et al.* (2013) Interests in high-functioning autism are more intense, interfering, and idiosyncratic than those in neurotypicals development. *Development and Psychopathology 25*, 3, 643–652.

APA (1980) *Diagnostic and Statistical Manual of Mental Disorders* (3rd Edition). Washington, DC: American Psychiatric Association.

APA (1994) *Diagnostic and Statistical Manual of Mental Disorders* (4th Edition). Washington, DC: American Psychiatric Association.

APA (2013) *Diagnostic and Statistical Manual of Mental Disorders* (5th Edition). Washington, DC: American Psychiatric Association.

Aral, A., Say, G.N. and Usta, M.B. (2018) Distinguishing circumscribed behavior in an adolescent with Asperger Syndrome from a pedophilic act: a case report. *Dusuren Adams – The Journal of Psychiatry and Neurological Sciences 31*, 1, 102.

Asperger, H. (1944) Autistichen Psychopathen in Kindersalter (Autistic psychopathy in childhood). *Archive fur Psychiatrie und Nevernkrankheiten 117*, 76–136.

Attwood, T. (1998) *Asperger's Syndrome: A Guide for Parents and Professionals*. London: Jessica Kingsley Publishers.

Audras-Torrent, L., Miniarikova, E., Couty, F., Dellapiazza, F. *et al.* (2021) WISC V profiles and their correlates in children with Autism Spectrum Disorder without Intellectual Development Disorder: report from the ELENA cohort. *Autism Research 14*, 5, 997–1006.

Autism Eye (2018) Parents vulnerable to FII allegations. www.autismeye.com/fabricated

Autistica (2017) Personal Tragedies, Public Crisis: The Urgent Need for a National Response to Early Death in Autism. www.autismeurope.org/wp-content/uploads/2017/08/personal-tragedies-public-crisis.pdf

Baio, J., Wiggins, L., Christensen, D.L., Maenner, M.J. *et al.* (2018) Prevalence of autism spectrum disorder among children aged 8 years – Autism and Developmental Disabilities Monitoring Network, 11 sites, United States, 2014. *Surveillance Summaries* 67, 6, 1–23. https://doi.org/10.15585/mmwr.ss6706a1

Bargiela, S., Steward, R. and Mandy, W. (2016) The experiences of late diagnosed women with Autism Spectrum Conditions: an investigation into the female Autism phenotype. *Journal of Autism and Developmental Disorders 46*, 3281–3294.

Baron-Cohen, S. (2002) The extreme male brain theory of autism. *Trends Cognitive Science 6*, 6, 248–254. doi: 10.1016/s1364-6613(02)01904-6. PMID: 12039606.

Baron-Cohen, S., Scott, F.J., Allison, C., Williams, J. *et al.* (2009) Prevalence of autism-spectrum conditions: UK school-based population study. *The British Journal of Psychiatry 194*, 6, 500–509. doi: 10.1192/bjp.bp.108.059345

Berryessa, C.M. (2016) Brief report: judicial attitudes regarding the sentencing of offenders with High Functioning Autism. *Journal of Autism and Developmental Disorders 46*, 8, 2770–2773.

Birmingham City Council (2011) *Adults with Autism and the Criminal Justice System: A Report from Overview & Scrutiny*. Birmingham: Birmingham City Council.

Bishop, S., Gahagan, S. and Lord, C. (2007) Re-examining the core features of autism: a comparison of ASD and FASD. *The Journal of Child Psychology and Psychiatry, and Allied Disciplines 48*, 11, 1111–1121.

Blackmore, C.E., Woodhouse, E.L., Gillan, N., Wilson, E. *et al.* (2022) Adults with autism spectrum disorder and the criminal justice system: an investigation of prevalence of contact with the criminal justice system, risk factors and sex differences in a specialist assessment service. *Autism 26*, 8. https://doi.org/10.1177/13623613221081343

Blakemore, M. (2015) Human Rights violations against parents that are Autistic, have an Autism Spectrum Condition, United Kingdom Human Rights Committee. https://abridgetoofartobefairtofermanagh.files.wordpress.com/2019/02/autism-human-rights-violations-against-parents-that-are-autistic-and-have-autism-spectrum-condition-.pdf

Bodner, E., Shriva, A., Hemesh, H., Ben-Ezra, M. and Iancu, I. (2015) Psychiatrists' fear of death is associated with negative emotions towards BPD patients. *Psychiatry Research 228*, 3, 963–965.

Bowlby, J. (1988) *A Secure Base: Parent and Child Attachment and Healthy Human Development*. New York: Basic Books.

Brewer, N. and Young, R.L. (2018) 'Interactions of Individuals with Autism Spectrum Disorder with the Criminal Justice System: Influences on Involvement and Outcomes.' In J.L. Johnson, G.S. Goodman and P.C. Mundy (eds) *The Wiley Handbook of Memory, Autism Spectrum Disorder and the Law*. Chichester: John Wiley & Sons. https://doi.org/10.1002/9781119158431.ch12

Cage, E. and Troxell-Whitman, Z. (2019) Understanding the reasons, contexts and costs of camouflaging for autistic adults. *Journal of Autism and Developmental Disorders 49*, 1899–1911.

Chapman, J., Jamil, R.T. and Fleister, C. (2022) Borderline Personality Disorder, in *Stat Pearls* [internet]. Treasure Island (FL): Stat Pearls Publishing. www.ncbi.nlm.nih.gov/books/NBK430883

Chisholm, T. and Coulter, A. (2017) Safeguarding and radicalisation. Research report. Department for Education. https://assets.publishing.service.gov.uk/government/uploads/system/uploads/attachment_data/file/635262/Safeguarding_and_Radicalisation.pdf

Choy, A. (1990) The Winner's Triangle. *Transactional Analysis Journal 20*, 1, 40–46.

Clarkson, P. (1987) The Bystander Role. *Transactional Analysis Journal 17*, 3, 82–87.

Clark, T., Feehan, C., Tinline, C. and Vostanis, P. (1999) Autistic symptoms in children with attention deficit-hyperactivity disorder. *European Child & Adolescent Psychiatry 8*, 50–55.

Colby, J. (2014) False allegations of child abuse in cases of myalgic encephalitis (ME). *Argument and Critique*, July.

Collins Dictionary (2022) Definition of vexatious. www.collinsdictionary.com/dictionary/english/vexatious

Corner, E. and Gill, P. (2017) Is there a nexus between terrorist involvement and mental health in the age of Islamic State? *CTC Sentinel 10*, 1, 1–11. https://ctc.westpoint.edu/wp-content/uploads/2017/01/CTC-Sentinel_Vol9Iss1121.pdf

Corner, E., Gill, P. and Mason, O. (2016) Mental health disorders and the terrorist: a research note probing selection effects and disorder prevalence. *Studies in Conflict and Terrorism 39*, 6, 560–568. https://doi.org/10.1080/1057610X.2015.1120099

Cridland, E.K., Jones, S.C., Caputi, P. and Magee, C.A. (2014) Being a girl in a boys' world: investigating the experiences of girls with autism spectrum disorders during adolescence. *Journal of Autism and Developmental Disorders 44*, 6, 1261–1274.

Crowell, S.C., Beauchaine, T.P. and Linehan, M.M. (2009) Elaborating and extending Linehan's theory. *Psychological Bulletin 135*, 3, 495–510.

Davidson, J.R.T., Hughes, D., Blazer, D.J. and George, L.K. (1991) Post-traumatic stress disorder in the community: an epidemiological study. *Psychological Medicine 21*, 3, 713–721.

Davis, P., Murtagh, V. and Glaser, D. (2019) 40 years of fabricated or induced illness (FII). Where next for paediatricians? Paper 1: Epidemiology and definition of FII. *Archives of Disease in Childhood 104*, 2, 110–114.

DCSF (Department for Children, Schools and Families) (2008) Department for Children, Schools and Families departmental report 2008. www.gov.uk/government/publications/department-for-children-schools-and-families-departmental-report-2008

De Berardis, D., Fornaro, M., Orsolini, L., Valchera, A. *et al.* (2017) Alexithymia and suicide risk in psychiatric disorders: a mini-review. *Frontiers in Psychiatry 8*, 148, 1–6.

Department of Health (2000) Framework for the Assessment of Children in Need and Their Families. https://bettercarenetwork.org/sites/default/files/Framework%20for%20othe%20Assessment%20of%20Children%20in%20Need%20and%20Their%20Families%20-%20Guidance%20Notes%20and%20Glossary.pdf

Desrosiers, L. (2015) Autism and Child Arrangement Disputes. www.familylawweek.co.uk/articles/autism-and-child-arrangement-disputes

DHSC MHA (1983, updated 2015 and 2017) Code of Practice: Mental Health Act 1983. www.gov.uk/government/publications/code-of-practice-mental-health-act-1983

Douglas, K.S., Shaffer, C., Blanchard, A.J.E., Guy, L.S., Reeves, K. and Weir, J. (2014) HCR-20 violence risk assessment scheme: overview and annotated bibliography. HCR-20 Violence Risk Assessment White Paper Series, #1. Burnaby, Canada: Mental Health, Law, and Policy Institute, Simon Fraser University.

Eaton, J. (2017) *A Guide to Mental Health Issues in Girls and Young Women on the Autism Spectrum: Diagnosis, Intervention and Support.* London: Jessica Kingsley Publishers.

Eaton, J. and Weaver, K. (2020) An exploration of the Pathological (or Extreme) Demand Avoidant profile in children referred for an autism diagnostic assessment using data from ADOS-2 assessments and from their developmental histories. *Good Autism Practice 21*, 2, 33–51.

Ehlers-Danlos Society (n.d.) Child Protection, EDS and HSD. www.ehlers-danlos.com/child-protection-and-eds

Eichner, M. (2015) 'The new child abuse panic.' *The New York Times*, 11 July 2015.

Esan, F., Chester, V., Gunaratna, I.J., Hoare, S. and Alexander, R.T. (2014) The clinical, forensic and treatment outcome factors of patients with autism spectrum disorder treated in a forensic intellectual disability service. *Journal of Applied Research in Intellectual Disabilities 28*, 3, 193–200.

Embracing Complexity (2022) Embracing Complexity in Diagnosis: Multi-Diagnostic Pathways for Neurodevelopmental Conditions. www.autistica.org.uk/downloads/files/Embracing-Complexity-in-Diagnosis.pdf

Faccini, L. and Allely, C. (2021) Dealing with trauma in individuals with Autism Spectrum Disorders: trauma informed care, treatment and forensic implications. *Journal of Aggression, Maltreatment and Trauma 30*, 8, 1082–1092.

Fernandes, L.C., Gillberg, C.I., Cederlund, M., Hagberg, B., Gillberg, C. and Billsted, E. (2016) Aspects of sexuality in adolescents and adults diagnosed with autism spectrum disorders in childhood. *Journal of Autism and Developmental Disorders 46*, 9, 3155–3165.

Fiightback (2019) False accusations of FII: a report by fiightback – March 2019. FIIGHTBACK.

Fombonne, E. (2009) Epidemiology of pervasive developmental disorders. *Pediatric Research 65*, 591–598.

Fonagy, P., Luyten, P., Allison, E. and Campbell, C. (2017) What we have changed our minds about: Part 1. Borderline Personality Disorder as a limitation of resilience. *Borderline Personality Disorder and Emotional Dysregulation 27*, 4, 11.

Forsyth, A. (2007) The effects of diagnosis and non-compliance attributions on therapeutic alliance in adult psychiatric settings. *Journal of Psychiatric and Mental Health Nursing 14*, 1, 33–40.

Fraser, K. and Gallop, R. (1993) Nurses' confirming/disconfirming responses to patients diagnosed with borderline personality disorder. *Archives of Psychiatric Nursing 7*, 6, 336–341.

Frick, P.J., Ray, J.V., Thornton, L.C. and Kahn, R.A. (2014) Annual Research Review: a developmental psychopathology approach to understanding callous-unemotional traits in children and adolescents with severe conduct problems. *Journal of Child Psychology and Psychiatry 55*, 6, 532–548.

Ghazziuden, M. (2005) *Mental Health Aspects of Autism and Asperger Syndrome*. London: Jessica Kingsley Publishers.

Gillberg, C. and Wing, L. (2007) Autism: not an extremely rare disorder. *Acta Psychiatrica Scandinavica 99*, 6, 399–406. https://doi.org/10.1111/j.1600-0447.1999.tb00984.x

Gotham, K., Risi, S., Pickles, A. and Lord, C. (2006) The Autism Diagnostic Observation Schedule (ADOS): revised algorithms for improved diagnostic diversity. *Journal of Autism and Developmental Disorders 37*, 4, 613–627.

Green, J., Absoud, M., Graham, V., Osman, M. *et al.* (2018) Pathological Demand Avoidance: symptoms but not a syndrome. *The Lancet Child & Adolescent Health 2*, 6, 455–464.

Green, R.M., Travers, A.M., Howe, Y. and McDouglas, C.J. (2019) Women and autism spectrum disorder: diagnosis and implications. *Current Psychiatry Reports 21*, 22. https://doi.org/10.1007/s11920-019-1006-3

Guerts, H.M. and Jansen, M.D. (2012) A retrospective chart study: the pathway to diagnosis for adults referred for ASD assessment. *Autism 16*, 3, 299–305.

Harvey, K. (2012) *Trauma-Informed Behavioral Interventions: What Works and What Doesn't.* Silver Springs, FL: American Association for Intellectual/Developmental Disabilities.

Hay, J. (1995) *Donkey Bridges for Developmental TA: Making Transactional Analysis Memorable and Accessible.* Hertford: Sherwood.

Hay, J. (2007) *Reflective Practice and Supervision for Coaches.* Maidenhead: Open University Press.

Hedley, D. and Uljarevic, M. (2018) Systematic review of suicide in Autism Spectrum Disorder: current trends and implications. *Current Developmental Disorders Reports* 5, 1, 65–76.

Heylens, G., Aspeslagh, L., Dierickx, J., Baetens, K. *et al.* (2018) The co-occurrence of gender dysphoria and autism spectrum disorder in adults: an analysis of cross-sectional and clinical chart data. *Journal of Autism and Developmental Disorders 48,* 6, 2217–2223.

Higgs, T. and Carter, A.J. (2015) Autism spectrum disorder and sexual offending: responsivity in forensic interventions. *Aggression and Violent Behavior 22,* May–June, 112–119.

HM Government (2008) Safeguarding Children in Whom Illness Is Fabricated or Induced. Supplementary guidance to working together to safeguard children. HM Government. www.londonsafeguardingchildrenprocedures.co.uk/files/sg_ch_fab_ill.pdf

Hobson, R.P. (1987) The autistic child's recognition of age- and sex-related characteristics of people. *Journal of Autism and Developmental Disorders 17,* 1, 63–79.

Hull, L., Petrides, K.V., Allison, C., Smith, P. *et al.* (2017) 'Putting on my best normal': social camouflaging in adults with autism spectrum conditions. *Journal of Autism and Developmental Disorders 47,* 8, 2519–2534.

Hussein, A. (2021) A participatory research approach to understanding the experiences of Black, Asian, and Minority Ethnic (BAME) Autistic young people. Thesis submitted for the degree of Professional Doctorate in Educational and Child Psychology. University of East London.

IACC (Interagency Autism Coordinating Committee) (2020) 2019 IACC Summary of Advances in Autism Spectrum Disorder Research. https://iacc.hhs.gov/publications/summary-of-advances/2019

itmustbemum (2017) It Must Be Mum – Part 4. *It Must Be Mum.* https://itmustbemum.wordpress.com/2017/02/03/it-must-be-mum-part-4

Johns Hopkins University (2020) U.S. autism rates up 10 percent in new CDC report. 20 July 2020. www.jhsph.edu/news/news-releases/2020/us-autism-rates-up-10-percent-in-new-cdc-report.html

Kandeh, S.M., Kandeh, K.M., Martin, N. and Krupa, J. (2020) Autism in Black, Asian and Minority Ethnic communities: a report on the first Autism Voice UK Symposium. *Advances in Autism 6,* 2, 165–175.

Kanner, L. (1943) 'Autistic disturbances of affective contact.' *Nervous Child: Journal of Psychopathology, Psychotherapy, Mental Hygiene, and Guidance of the Child 2,* 217–250.

Karpman, S. (1968) Fairy tales and script drama analysis. *Transactional Analysis Bulletin 7,* 26, 39–43.

Kendell, R.E. (2002) The distinction between personality disorder and mental illness. *British Journal of Psychiatry 180,* 110–115.

Kernberg, O.F. and Michels, R. (2009) Borderline Personality Disorder. *American Psychiatry 166*, 5, 505–508.

King, C. and Murphy, G.H. (2014) A systematic review of people with autism spectrum disorder and the criminal justice system. *Journal of Autism and Developmental Disorders 44*, 11, 2717–2733.

Kogan, M.D., Blumberg, S.J., Schieve, L.A., Boyle, C.A. *et al.* (2009) Prevalence of parent-reported diagnosis of autism spectrum disorder among children in the US, 2007. *Pediatrics 124*, 5, 1395–1403. doi: 10.1542/peds.2009-1522

Kolta, B. and Rossi, G. (2018) Paraphilic disorder in a male patient with autism spectrum disorder: incidence or coincidence. *Cureus 10*, 5, e2639. doi: 10.7759/cureus.2639

Kosatka, D. and Ona, C. (2014) Eye movement desensitization and reprocessing in a patient with Asperger's disorder: case report. *Journal of EMDR Practice and Research 8*, 1, 13–18. https://doi.org/10.1891/1933-3196.8.1.13

Kreiser, N.L. and White, S.W. (2014) ASD in females: are we overstating the gender difference in diagnosis? *Clinical Child Family Psychological Review 17*, 1, 67–84.

Långström, N., Grann, M., Ruchkin, V., Sjöstedt, G. and Fazel, S. (2009) Risk factors for violent offending in autism spectrum disorder: a national study of hospitalized individuals. *Journal of Interpersonal Violence 24*, 8, 1358–1370. doi: 10.1177/0886260508322195

Lavigne, J.V., Bryant, F.B., Hopkins, J. and Gouze, K.R. (2015) Dimensions of oppositional defiance disorder in young children: model comparisons, gender and longitudinal invariance. *Journal of Abnormal Child Psychology 43*, 3, 423–439.

Leichsenring, F., Leibing, E., Kruse, J., New, A.S. and Leweke, F. (2011) Borderline Personality Disorder. *Lancet 377*, 74–84.

Lindsay, W., Carson, D., O'Brian, G., Holland, A. *et al.* (2014) A comparison of referrals with and without autism spectrum disorder to forensic intellectual disability services. *Psychiatry, Psychology and Law 21*, 6, 947–954.

London Borough of Southwark (2016) London Borough of Southwark Safeguarding Service Parenting Assessment Framework, Practitioner Handbook. Guidance for social workers undertaking assessments of parenting capacity. https://southwark.proceduresonline.com/pdfs/parent_assess.pdf

Long, C., Eaton, J., Russell, S., Gullen-Scott, F. and Bilson, A. (2022) Fabricated or Induced Illness and Perplexing Presentations: Abbreviated Practice Guide for Social Work Practitioners. Birmingham: BASW. www.basw.co.uk/resources/fabricated-and-induced-illness-practice-guide

Lord, C., Rutter, M. and LeCouteur, A. (1994) Autism Diagnostic Interview – Revised: a revised version of a diagnostic interview for caregivers of individuals with possible pervasive developmental disorders. *Journal of Autism and Developmental Disorders 24*, 5, 659–685.

Lovelace, T.S., Cornis, M.P., Tabb, J.V. and Oshokoya, O.E. (2021) Missing from the narrative: a seven-decade scoping review of the inclusion of Black autistic women and girls in autism research. *Behavior Analysis in Practice 15*, 1093–1105. https://doi.org/10.1007/s40617-021-00654-9

Mademtzi, M., Singh, P., Shic, F. and Koenig, K. (2018) Challenges of females with autism: a parental perspective. *Journal of Autism and Developmental Disorders 48*, 4, 1301–1310.

Maenner, M.J., Shaw, K.A., Baio, J., Washington, A. *et al.* (2020) Prevalence of autism spectrum disorder among children aged 8 years—Autism and Developmental

Disabilities Behavior Analysis Practice Monitoring Network, 11 sites, United States, 2016. *Surveillance Summaries 69*, 4, 1–12. https://doi.org/10.15585/mmwr.ss6904a1

Mandell, D.S., Ittenbach, R.F., Levy, S.E. and Pinto-Martin, J.A. (2007) Disparities in diagnoses received prior to a diagnosis of autism spectrum disorder. *Journal of Autism and Developmental Disorders 37*, 9, 1795–1802.

Mandell, D.S., Walrath, C.M., Manteuffel, B., Sgro, G. and Pinto Martin, J.A. (2005) The prevalence and correlates of abuse among children with autism served in comprehensive community-based mental health settings. *Child Abuse & Neglect 29*, 12, 1359–1372.

Mandy, W. (2019) Social camouflaging in autism: is it time to lose the mask? *Autism 23*, 8, 1879–1881.

Maras, K.L., Crane, L., Mulcahy, S., Hawken, T. *et al.* (2017) Brief report: autism in the courtroom: experiences of legal professionals and the autism community. *Journal of Autism and Developmental Disorders 47*, 8, 2610–2620.

Markham, D. and Trower, P. (2003) The effects of the psychiatric label 'borderline personality disorder' on nursing staff's perceptions and casual attributions for challenging behaviours. *The British Journal of Clinical Psychology 42*, 3, 243–256.

Martin, N. and Milton, D. (2017) 'Supporting the Inclusion of Autistic Children.' In G. Knowles (ed.) *Supporting Inclusive Practice and Ensuring Opportunity Is Equal for All*. Abingdon: David Fulton, Routledge.

Mason, D., Stewart, G.R., Capp, S.J. and Happe, F. (2022) Older age autism research: a rapidly growing field but still a long way to go. *Autism in Adulthood 4*, 2, 164–172.

Matson, J.L., Rieske, R.D. and Williams, L.W. (2013) The relationship between autism spectrum disorders and attention-deficit/hyperactivity disorder: an overview. *Research in Developmental Disabilities 34*, 9, 2475–2484.

Matthys, W. and Lochman, J.E. (2017) *Oppositional Defiant Disorder and Conduct Disorder in Childhood*, 2nd edn. Chichester, New York: John Wiley & Sons.

May, T., Pilkington, P.D., Younan, R. and Williams, K. (2021) Overlap of autism spectrum disorder and borderline personality disorder: a systematic review and meta-analysis. *Autism Research 14*, 12, 2688–2710.

McClure, R.J., Davis, P.M. and Meadow, S.R. (1996) Epidemiology of Munchausen syndrome by proxy: non-accidental poisoning and non-accidental suffocation. *Archives of Disease in Childhood 75*, 1, 57–61.

Meadow, R. (1977) Munchausen syndrome by proxy. The hinterland of child abuse. *Lancet 2*, 8033, 343–345.

Meadow, R. (1982) Munchausen syndrome by proxy. *Archives of Disease in Childhood 57*, 2, 92–98.

Meadow, R. (1995) What is, and what is not, 'Munchausen syndrome by proxy'. *Archives of Disease in Childhood 72*, 6, 534–538.

Milton, D.E.M. (2012) On the ontological status of autism: the double empathy problem. *Disability and Society 27*, 6, 883–887.

Mogavero, M.C. (2016) Autism, sexual offending and the criminal justice system. *Journal of Intellectual Disabilities and Offending Behaviour 7*, 116–126. doi: 10.1108/JIDOB-02-2016-0004

Mouridsen, S.E. (2012) Current status of research on autism spectrum disorders and offending. *Research in Autism Spectrum Disorders 6*, 1, 79–86.

Murphy, D. (2013) Risk assessment of offenders with an autism spectrum disorder. *Journal of Intellectual Disabilities and Offending Behaviour 4*, 1–2, 33–41.

NAS (National Autistic Society) (2011) *Autism: A Guide for Criminal Justice Professionals*. London: National Autistic Society.

NAS (National Autistic Society) (2022) Number of autistic people in mental health hospitals. 17th February 2022. www.autism.org.uk/what-we-do/news/autistic-people-in-mental-health-hospitals

Newson, E. (1983) Pathological demand-avoidance syndrome. *Communication 17*, 3–8.

Newson, E., LeMarechal, K. and David, C. (2003) Pathological demand avoidance syndrome: a necessary distinction within the pervasive developmental disorders. *Archives of Disease in Childhood 88*, 7, 595–600.

NHS (n.d.) Overview – Fabricated or induced illness. www.nhs.uk/mental-health/conditions/fabricated-or-induced-illness/overview

NICE (2017) Autism spectrum disorder in under 19s: recognition, referral and diagnosis. Clinical Guidance [CG128]. www.nice.org.uk/guidance/cg128

Not Fine in School (2018) School attendance difficulties: Parent survey results NOT Fine in School. https://notfineinschool.co.uk/nfis-surveys

O'Nions, E., Viding, E., Greven, C.U., Ronald, A. and Happé, F. (2014) Pathological demand avoidance: exploring the behavioural profile. *Autism 18*, 5, 538–544.

PANDAS/PANS UK (2022) PANDAS/PANS. www.pandasuk.org

Parent and Carer Alliance (2019) The impact of FII allegations on parents – report summary. www.parentandcareralliance.org.uk/wp-content/uploads/2019/03/PCA-FII-Summary-final-shared.pdf

PDA Society (2022, January) Identifying & Assessing a PDA Profile – Practice Guidance. www.pdasociety.org.uk/resources/identifying-assessing-a-pda-profile-practice-guidance

Pierce, N.P., O'Reilly, M.F., Sorrells, A.M., Fragale, C.L. *et al.* (2014) Ethnicity reporting practices for empirical research in three autism-related journals. *Journal of Autism & Developmental Disorders 44*, 7, 1507–1519. https://doi.org/10.1007/s10803-014-2041-x

Plotnikoff, J. and Woolfson, R. (2015) *Intermediaries in the Criminal Justice System: Improving Communication for Vulnerable Witnesses and Defendants*. Bristol: Policy Press.

Pohl, A.L., Crockford, S.K., Blakemore, M., Allison, C. and Baron-Cohen, S. (2020) A comprehensive study of autistic and non-autistic women's experience of motherhood. *Molecular Autism 11*, 3. https://doi.org/10.1186/s13229-019-0304-2

Ramclam, A.N., Truong, D.M., Mire, S.S., Smoots, K.D. *et al.* (2022) Autism disparities for black children: acknowledging and addressing the problem through culturally responsive and socially just assessment practices. *Psychology in the Schools 59*, 1445–1453.

RCPCH (2002) *Fabricated or Induced Illness by Carers. Royal College of Paediatrics and Child Health*. London: RCPCH.

RCPCH (2009) *Fabricated or Induced Illness by Carers (FII): A Practical Guide for Paediatricians*. London: RCPCH.

RCPCH (2021) Perplexing Presentations (PP)/Fabricated or Induced Illness in Children – Guidance. https://childprotection.rcpch.ac.uk/resources/perplexing-presentations-and-fii

Ring, D. and Lawn, S. (2019) Stigma perpetuation and the interface of mental health care: a review to compare patient and clinical perspectives of stigma and borderline personality disorder. *Journal of Mental Health 12*, 12–21. doi: 10.1080/09638237.1581537

Roberts, G. (2006) 'Disgraced Meadow reinstated by judge.' *Independent*, 18 February 2006. www.independent.co.uk/news/uk/crime/disgraced-meadow-reinstated-by-judge-346182.html

Rogers, G., Rogers, L., Ukoumunne, O. and Ford, T. (2014) Prevalence of parent-reported ASD and ADHD in the UK: findings from the Millennium Cohort Study. *Journal of Autism and Developmental Disorders 44*, 1, 31–40.

Rommelse, N.N., Franke, B., Geurts, H.M., Hartman, C.A. and Buitelaar, J.K. (2010) Shared heritability of attention-deficit/hyperactivity disorder and autism spectrum disorder. *European Child & Adolescent Psychiatry 19*, 3, 281–295.

Rommelse, N.N., Geurts, H.M., Franke, B., Buitelaar, J.K. and Hartman, C.A. (2011) A review on cognitive and brain endophenotypes that may be common in autism spectrum disorder and attention-deficit/hyperactivity disorder and facilitate the search for pleiotropic genes. *Neuroscience & Biobehavioral Reviews 35*, 6, 1363–1396.

Ronald, A., Simonoff, E., Kuntsi, J., Asherson, P. and Plomin, R. (2008) Evidence for overlapping genetic influences on autistic and ADHD behaviours in a community twin sample. *Journal of Child Psychology and Psychiatry and Allied Disciplines 49*, 5, 535–554.

Royal College of Psychiatrists (2014) Good practice in the management of autism (including Asperger syndrome) in adults. Royal College of Psychiatrists, London. www.rcpsych.ac.uk/usefulresources/publications/collegereports/cr/cr191.aspx

Royal College of Psychiatrists (2020) The psychiatric management of autism in adults. www.rcpsych.ac.uk/improving-care/campaigning-for-better-mental-health-policy/college-reports/2020-college-reports/cr228

Russell, P. and Kelly, S. (2011) Looking beyond risk: a study of lay epidemiology of childhood disorders. *Health, Risk & Society 13*, 2, 129.

Sackett, D.L. (1997) Evidence based medicine. *Seminars in Perinatology 21*, 1, 3–5. doi: 10.1016/s0146-0005(97)80013-4

Scottish Executive Social Research (2004) *On the Borderline? People with Learning Disabilities and/or Autistic Spectrum Disorders in Secure, Forensic and Other Specialist Settings.* Scottish Executive Social Research: Edinburgh.

Scragg, P. and Shah, A. (1994) Prevalence of Asperger's syndrome in a secure hospital. *British Journal of Psychiatry 165*, 5, 679–682.

Secretary of State Case Review (2019) Secretary of State Case Review into Beth. https://assets.publishing.service.gov.uk/government/uploads/system/uploads/attachment_data/file/845670/Serious_incident_investigation_report_-_Secretary_of_State_case_review_into_Beth.pdf

Sheridan, M.S. (2003) The deceit continues: an updated literature review of Munchausen syndrome by proxy. *Child Abuse & Neglect 27*, 4, 431–451.

Shine, J. and Cooper-Evans, S. (2016) Developing an autism specific framework for forensic case formulation. *Journal of Intellectual Disabilities and Offending Behaviour 7*, 3, 127–139. https://doi.org/10.1108/JIDOB-04-2015-0006

Siret, D. (2019) An examination of Fabricated and Induced Illness cases in Gloucestershire. A report from the Parent and Carer Alliance C.I.C. Parent and Carer Alliance. www.parentandcareralliance.org.uk/wp-content/uploads/2019/03/PCA-FII-Summary-final-shared.pdf

Slade, G. (2014) *Diverse Perspectives: The Challenges for Families Affected by Autism from Black, Asian and Minority Ethnic Communities.* London: The National Autistic Society.

Social Work England (2020) Working Together to Safeguard Children (updated July 2022). www.workingtogetheronline.co.uk

Sokolova, E., Oerlemans, A.M. and Rommelse, N.N. (2017). A causal and mediation analysis of the comorbidity between attention deficit hyperactivity disorder

(ADHD) and autism spectrum disorder (ASD). *Journal of Autism & Developmental Disorders 47*, 6, 1595–1604. https://doi.org/10.1007/s10803-017-3083-7

Stewart, I. and Joines, V. (2012) *TA Today: A New Introduction to Transactional Analysis*, 2nd edn. Chapel Hill, NC: Lifespace Publishing.

Stokes, M.A. and Kaur, A. (2005) High functioning autism and sexuality: a parental perspective. *Autism 9*, 3, 266–289.

Straiton, D. and Sridhar, A. (2022) Short Report: call to action for autism clinicians in response to anti-Black racism. *Autism 26*, 4, 988–994.

Strang, J.F., Janssen, A., Tishelman, A., Leibowitz, S.F. *et al.* (2018a) Revisiting the link: evidence of the rates of autism in studies of gender diverse individuals. *Journal of the American Academy of Child and Adolescent Psychiatry 57*, 11, 885–886.

Strang, J.F., Meagher, H., Kenworthy, L., De Vries, A.L.C. *et al.* (2018b) Initial clinical guidelines for co-occurring autism spectrum disorder and gender dysphoria or incongruence in adolescents. *Journal of Clinical Child & Adolescent Psychology 47*, 1, 105–115.

Sulzer, S.H. (2015) Does 'difficult patient' status contribute to de facto de-medicalisation? The case of borderline personality disorder. *Social Science and Medicine 142*, 82–89.

Tantam, D. (2012) *Autism Spectrum Disorders through the Lifespan*. London: Jessica Kingsley Publishers.

Tarren-Sweeney, M. (2013) An investigation of complex attachment and trauma-related symptomatology among children in foster and kinship care. *Child Psychiatry and Human Development 44*, 6, 727–741.

Turban, J.L. and van Schalkwyk, G.I. (2018) Gender dysphoria and autism spectrum disorder: is the link real? *Journal of the American Academy of Child and Adolescent Psychiatry 57*, 8–9, e2.

Van der Kolk, B.A. (2005) Developmental trauma disorder: toward a rational diagnosis for children with complex trauma histories. *Psychiatric Annals 35*, 5, 401–408.

Van der Kolk, B.A., Pynoos, R.S., Cicetti, D., Cloitre, M. *et al.* (2009) Proposal to include a developmental trauma diagnosis for children and adolescents in DSM 5. www.complextrauma.org/wp-content/uploads/2019/03/Complex-Trauma-Resource-3-Joseph-Spinazzola.pdf

Walter, F., Leonard, S., Miah, S. and Shaw, J. (2021) Characteristics of autism spectrum disorder and susceptibility to radicalism among young people: a qualitative study. *The Journal of Forensic Psychiatry and Psychology 32*, 3, 408–429.

Weight, E.J. and Kendal, S. (2013) Staff attitudes towards inpatients with borderline personality disorder. *Mental Health Practice 17*, 3, 34–38.

Welsh Assembly Government (2008) Safeguarding Children in Whom Illness is Fabricated or Induced. www.cysur.wales/media/grofqaa3/safeguarding_children_in_whom_illness_is_fabricated_or_induced.pdf

Went, H.E. (2016) I didn't fit the stereotype of autism: a qualitative analysis of women's experiences relating to diagnosis of an Autism Spectrum Condition and mental health. Thesis submitted as part fulfilment for the degree of Doctor of Clinical Psychology. University of Exeter.

Zaroff, C.M. and Uhm, S.Y. (2011) Prevalence of autism spectrum disorders and influence of country of measurement and ethnicity. *Social Psychiatry and Psychiatric Epidemiology 47*, 3, 395–398. doi: 10.1007/s00127-011-0350-3

Subject Index

Author Index